25 Secrets of Tai Chi

Original Title

'Chen Family Taijiquan 25 Key Disciplines'

(陳氏太極拳 二十五 練拳秘訣)

Advisor: Chen Bing

Author: Bosco Baek

Editor: Daniel Iorio, Christopher Wang, Sasan Jahan-Parwar

Revised Edition

This revised edition was corrected to add more information for clarification and easier understanding. This book would be just difficult to comprehend proverbs if you learned only the external forms of Taijiquan. If you have great instruction that provides the internal principles of Taijiquan, this book will become your Taiji bible to enlighten you. The second edition was completed on July 18 Tuesday 2017.

Contents (目次)

List of 25 Key Disciplines in Chinese   p. 5

List of 25 Key Disciplines in English   p. 6

Tai Chi or Taijiquan?   P. 7

About the Author   p. 8

Preface by Chen Bing   p. 12

Preface by Bosco Baek   p. 15

Introduction to Annotation of Chen Family Taijiquan 25 Key Disciplines   p. 18

What is 'Fang Song'?   p. 20

The Law of Body   p. 23

The Law of Mind   p. 61

The Law of Reeling Silk   p. 88

4 Major Characteristics   p. 111

General Terms in Chinese Culture   p. 127

General Terms in Western Culture   p. 133

Chen Family Taijiquan Tree of Bosco Baek in USA   p. 135

Additional writing by Bosco Baek   p. 139

Chen Family Taijiquan 25 Key Disciplines
陳氏太極拳 二十五 練拳秘訣

The Law of Body （身法：shēn fǎ）

1. 虛領頂勁　　Xū Lǐng Dǐng Jìn
2. 鬆肩沈肘　　Sōng Jiān Chén Zhǒu
3. 含胸塌腰，　Hán Xiōng Tā Yāo,
   尾閭中正　　Wěi Lú Zhōng Zhèng
4. 屈膝鬆胯　　Qū Xī Sōng Kuà
5. 垂臀圓襠　　Chuí Tún Yuán Dāng
6. 下盘稳固　　Xià Pán Wěn Gù
7. 立身中正　　Lì Shēn Zhōng Zhèng
8. 上虛下實，　Shàng Xū Xià Shí,
   虛實分明　　Xū Shí Fēn Míng
9. 八面支撐　　Bā Miàn Zhī Chēng

The Law of Mind （心法：xīn fǎ）

10. 全身放鬆　　Quán Shēn Fàng Sōng
11. 心氣下降　　Xīn Qì Xià Jiàng
12. 意守丹田，　Yì Shǒu Dān Tián,
    氣沈丹田　　Qì Chén Dān Tián
13. 感受呼吸　　Gǎn Shòu Hū Xī
14. 氣貫周身　　Qì Guàn Zhōu Shēn
15. 不丟不頂　　Bù Diū Bù Dǐng

The Law of Reeling Silk （纏絲法：chán sī fǎ）

16. 以腰爲軸　　Yǐ Yāo Wéi Zhóu
17. 胸腰折疊　　Xiōng Yāo Zhé Dié
18. 丹田運轉　　Dān Tián Yùn Zhuǎn
19. 節節貫串　　Jié Jié Guàn Chuàn
20. 意到氣到，　Yì Dào Qì Dào,
    氣到形到　　Qì Dào Xíng Dào
21. 內外相合，　Nèi Wài Xiāng Hé,
    周身一家　　Zhōu Shēn Yì Jiā

The 4 Major Characteristics （四大特點：sì dà tè diǎn）

22. 剛柔并(相)濟，Gāng Róu Bīng (Xiàng) Jǐ,
    快慢相間　　Kuài Màn Xiāng Jiàn
23. 蓄發相變　　Xù Fā Xiāng Biàn
24. 鬆活彈抖　　Sōng Huó Tán Dǒu
25. 外形走弧線，Wài Xíng Zǒu Hú Xiàn,
    內勁走旋　　Nèi Jìn Zǒu Luó Xuán

Chen Family Taijiquan 25 Key Disciplines
from direct translations
The Law of Body （身法：shēn fǎ）

1. Make the crown of the head empty and upright.
2. Loosen up the shoulder and immerge the elbow.
3. Incubate the chest and suspend the lower back.
   The door of the tail is centered and upright.
4. Bend the knees and relax the hip.
5. Hang the buttocks and round the groin.
6. Be comfortable and solid under a tray.
7. The body stands up in the center correctly.
8. The upper is empty and the lower is full.
   The empty and the full are clearly split.
9. Support in eight sides.

The Law of Mind （心法：xīnfǎ）

10. Relax the whole body deeply.
11. Go down the energy of mind to the low.
12. Protect dantian with intention.
    Sink energy into dantian.
13. Feel and take exhalation and inhalation.
14. Penetrate energy far through the body.
15. Not to be lost and greatly.

The Law of Reeling Silk （纏絲法：chán sī fǎ）

16. Use the waist as an axis
17. The chest and waist connect and fold.
18. Dantian rotates and moves.
19. Pass and penetrate through joint by joint.
20. Intention reaches and then energy reaches.
    Energy reaches and then shape reaches.
21. Combine in and out mutually.
    The body becomes evenly one house.

The 4 Major Characteristics （四大特點：sì dà tè diǎn）

22. Help the hard and soft mutually.
    Mix the fast and slow mutually.
23. Cultivating and discharging mutually change.
24. Be relaxed, alive, elastic and vibrating.
25. It goes in a circular line in an external form.
    The internal force rotates in a spiral line.

Tai Chi or Taijiquan?

Tai Chi (Tai Chi Chuan) is the phonetic spelling of the Chinese term, Taijiquan (太極拳 tàijíquán). Taijiquan is correct according to the Chinese Pinyin system. The correct pronunciation of Taijiquan is 'tai-ji-chuan'. It is also simply called Taiji.

Most foreigners use 'Tai Chi' broadly because it is simple to say and they are unclear how to pronounce the 'q' sound. It actually sounds like 'ch' in the Chinese Pinyin system.

Please use the accurate pronunciation of Taijiquan.

About the Author

Bosco Baek (白承哲 bái chéng zhé) is the sole Korean-American disciple of Master Chen Bing in the USA and a senior disciple of 'The Old Ten Disciples (十徒弟 lǎo shí túdì)' who were accepted by Master Chen Bing in 2004 and 2005. Master Baek is the head of the Chen Bing Taiji Academy USA in Los Angeles and teaches classical Chen Family Taijiquan as taught by Master Chen Bing in Chenjiagou. Master Baek is the first person to bring his teacher, Master Chen Bing, to the USA in 2004. In October 5th 2014, Master Bosco Baek was appointed an 'Excellent Successor of Chen Family Taijiquan (陈氏太极拳优秀传承人 chén shì tài jí quán yōu xiù chuán chéng rén)' by the Chen Village Committee and China Chen Village Taijiquan Association.

Born in April, 1978 in South Korea, Master Baek was raised in a Chinese branch of the Baek family (水原白氏 shuǐ yuán bái shì); 31st generation and eldest son of the Moon-Kyung Gong lineage (文敬公派 wén jìng gōngpài). In 1992, Master Baek started Chinese Hygiene Qigong at age 13 and studied classical Raja and Hatha Yoga from the Himalaya Meditation Center and Korea Yoga Academy in 1996. In 1999, he started Chen Family Taijiquan under Master Myung-Won Seo who is the first foreign disciple of

Grand Master Chen Xiaoxing. In 2000, he started learning from Master Chen Bing and became his formal disciple on Christmas day, 2005 in Chenjiagou. Master Baek is also an instructor of Chinese Hygiene Qigong (中華養生益智功 zhōnghuá yǎngshēng yìzhì gōng), Sva Sam Vidya Raja Yoga (स्व सम् विद्या, Himalaya Meditation Center), Anuka Yoga Cikitsa (अनूक योग चिकित्सा, Korea Yoga Academy), Svastha Yoga (स्वस्थ, A.G. Mohan), and a former Taiji Professor at Samra University. He graduated from Loyola University Chicago and majored in biology.

He now teaches the essence of Chen Family Taijiquan and his three yoga styles known as Ekatala Yoga. He is a particularly skilled expert at teaching and applying Taijiquan and Yoga therapy based on an individual student's need.

Master Baek currently runs the Chen Bing Taiji Academy USA (美國陳炳太極院 měiguó chén bǐng tàijí yuàn) in Los Angeles.

Certifications and Positions

1993 Chinese Hygiene Qigong Instructor (3rd level)

1999 Yoga Teacher at Korea Yoga Academy

2002 Yoga Teacher at Himalaya Meditation Center

2002 Certified Instructor at Chenjiagou Taijiquan School

2004 President of World Chen Family Taijiquan USA

2005 Advanced Instructor at Chen Village Martial Arts Association

2006 Svastha Yoga Instructor by A.G. Mohan

2008 President and head teacher of Chen Bing Taiji Academy USA

2014 Appointed 'Excellent Successor of Chen Family Taijiquan' by Chen Villagers Committee and the China Chen Village Taijiquan Association

2016 Certificate of Recognition by the California State Assembly

2016 Appointed 'Excellent Coach' by Chen Bing Taiji Academy Chenjiagou Headquarters

Medals and Awards

2002 6th Korea National Taijiquan Tournament; Gold Medal (Old Frame First Road), Silver Medal (New Frame First Road)

2004 Chicago International Wushu-Gongfu Tournament; Gold Medal (Old Frame First Road, Sword)

2008 Illinois Open Martial Arts Championship; Gold Medal (Old Frame, New Frame, Sword)

2009 Illinois Open Martial Arts Championship; Gold Medal (Old Frame, New Frame, Sword)

2015   The 8th China Jiaozuo International Taijiquan Exchange Competition; Silver Medal (Chen Family Taijiquan Single Straight Sword), Bronze Medal (Combined Complex Chen Family Taijiquan)

2016   24th Chinese Martial Arts Tournament (CMAT); Gold Medal (Advanced Taiji Spear, Advanced Straight Sword, Silver Medal (Advanced Combined Chen Taiij),Bronze Medal (Advanced Cannon Fist)

2017   2nd Chenjiagou Taijiquan Exchange Competition Gold Medal (Double Straight Sword), Bronze Medal (Single Straight Sword)

Other Contributions

2012   Nissan Altima TV advertisement (Chinese version)

2014   METRO Los Angeles Retreat Workshop

2015   FBI Los Angeles Branch Workshop

2015   Guinness World Records; Largest martial arts display (multiple venues)

Degree

B.S. in Biology (Loyola University Chicago)

Preface (序 xù) by Chen Bing

太极拳是17世纪人类的一项重大发明是中国武术发展的又一次飞跃是东方太极哲学思想的有形表现。它不仅使人在身体、武术技能上得到发展更会在精神、生命力以及人类智慧上得以修炼他是21世纪最完美的身心和谐运动。

Taijiquan is an important 17th century creation which was a leap in development of Chinese martial arts and a manifestation of Asian Taiji philosophy. Taijiquan makes us not only train the body and develop martial art skills, but also gain the spirit, vital force and wisdom of humankind. This is the perfect (完美 wán měi) harmony of uniting the body and mind to its peak in the 21st century.

白承哲曾多次到太极拳的发源地--
中国陈家沟学习太极拳考察它的历史脉络研究它的内在机理是太极拳运动的痴迷者和践行者。同时又拥有多年医学和瑜伽方面的知识和经验在美国开展太极拳专业教学也已经有十多年的时间了积累了大量的专业知识和实践经验是我比较欣赏和认可的徒弟之一。

Bosco Baek has practiced at the birth place of Taijiquan, Chen Village in China. He learned the history of Taijiquan, studied its internal principles, and became an enthusiast and practitioner of Taijiquan. He also possesses knowledge of medicine and yoga thanks to many years of practice. Furthermore, he has taught and practiced Taijiquan professionally for well over ten years, and has accumulated vast practical knowledge and teaching experience. He is a disciple of mine whom I appreciate and recognize.

将复杂的太极拳运动提炼凝结形成简单易学同时保留太极拳的真义并能使学者短时间内收获到太极拳的益处一直是我们的心愿这也是太极拳未来发展的一个趋势。
To extract the complicated disciplines of Taijiquan practices, to simplify them; to learn easily with clarification, but to have the essence (真义 zhēn yì) of Taijiquan simultaneously, while allowing practitioners to benefit in a short period of time is our long-time wish for the future development of Taijiquan.

因此在白承哲的努力下经过我们的不断实践和研究终于编写出了这部陈氏太极拳教程我相信这将是太极拳爱好者的福音也是陈氏太极拳发展史上的又一次美好历程。
Therefore, with the effort of Bosco Baek (白承哲) and our continuous practice and research, it is possible to finally publish the key disciplines of Chen Family Taijiquan. I believe that this is the gospel for Taijiquan enthusiasts and another wonderful development in Taijiquan history.

在此我向广大的读者、太极拳爱好者祝福向徒弟白承哲祝贺。也为陈氏太极拳能更多地造福人类而感到骄傲。

Hereby, I send blessings to the readers and enthusiasts of Taijiquan, and congratulate my disciple, Bosco Baek. Also, I am proud that Chen Family Taijiquan can benefit mankind.

January 14 2014

陈家沟国际太极院(陈炳太极院)院长 陈炳

President of Chen Bing Taiji Academy

Chen Bing (陈炳)

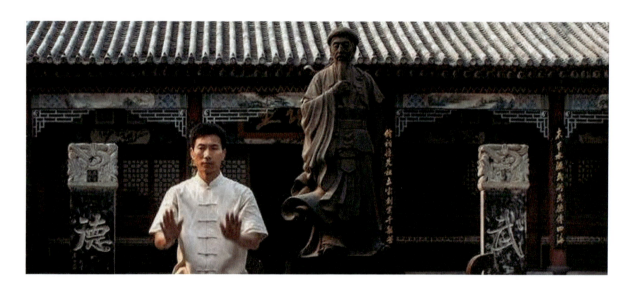

Master Chen Bing in front of the statue of Chen Wangting who is the Taijiquan creator at Chenjiagou - the birthplace of Taijiquan

Preface(序 xù) by Bosco Baek

Nowadays, there are many people who practice Taijiquan (太極拳 tài jí quán), however most of them believe that this simply involves practicing slow movements, without capturing the essence of proper Taijiquan study. The original and classical Taijiquan is not about mastering external forms. It is to physically learn (體得 tǐ dé) and consciously realize (心得 xīn dé) the key disciplines (要訣 yào jué) of Taijiquan.

It is no small feat to put these principles on paper, and I know that some are so subtle, that it will be difficult to clearly express. This is because it is simply better to physically realize and experience these key disciplines directly from a teacher. Just a few years ago, I thought only the chosen ones could learn these secrets. Frankly, I never wanted to open up or share them with anyone. However, my mind was changed by the tumultuous nature of this world and storms of my life. So these days, rather than being a lonely master (高手 gāoshǒu) of Taijiquan, I want to share the quintessence (眞髓 zhēnsuǐ) of Taijiquan with many people. With the permission of my Shifu (師父 shī fu), Chen Bing, it will be the first Chen Family Taijiquan 25 key disciplines as handed down from a direct descendant(嫡傳統 dí chuán tǒng)of Taijiquan's creator, Chen Wang Ting. Master Chen Bing hails from the birth place (發源地 fā yuándì) of

Taijiquan, Chenjiagou (aka Chen Village), Wenxian County, Henan Province, China (中國 zhōngguó 河南省 hénánshěng 溫縣 wēnxiàn 陳家溝 chénjiā gōu). I did my utmost to keep it simple and clear.

Chen Family Taijiquan, as transmitted by my Shifu, is the harmony (調和 tiáohé) and fusion (融和 rónghé) of Chinese medicine (中醫學 zhōngyīxué), internal power (內功 nèigōng), and martial arts (武術 wǔshù) which is marvelous (神妙 shénmiào) for well-being (健身 jiànshēn) and self defense (護身 hù shēn).

Do make a concerted effort to find a certified Chen Family Taijiquan instructor should this article spawn any interest. I sincerely hope that all practitioners gain the true essence of Taijiquan.

Furthermore, this annotation of key disciplines (要訣註解 yào jué zhù jiě) may become a text book not only for Chen Family Taijiquan practitioners, but also practitioners of other Taijiquan styles. I wish to develop all practitioners' understanding, and to improve the quality and depth of their practice.

Regards,

January 5 2014

President of Chen Bing Taiji Academy USA

Bosco Baek (白承哲)

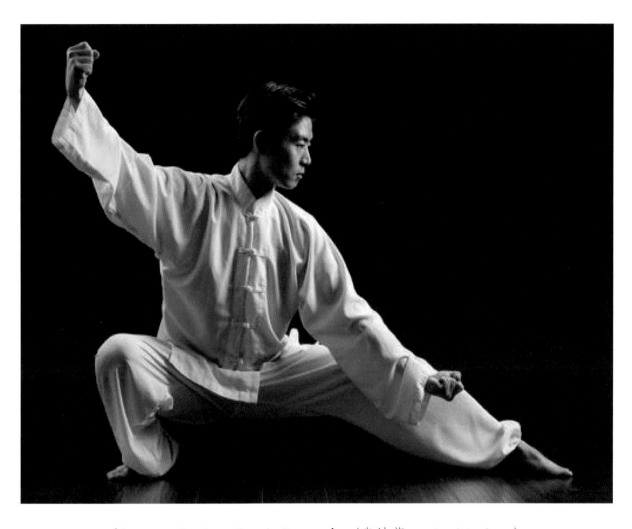

'Sparrow Dashes Earth Dragon' (雀地龍 què dì long)

in Old Frame First Road(架一路 lǎo jià yí lù)

photo by Christopher Soule in 2012

Introduction to Annotation (要訣註解 yào jué zhù jiě) of Chen Family Taijiquan 25 Key Disciplines

Before developing his own style (一家 yì jiā) of Taijiquan, Yang Lu Chan (楊露禪 yáng lù chán), founder of Yang Family Taijiquan, first learned the internal martial art from a 14th generation representative of the Chen family named Chen Chang Xing (陳長興 chén cháng xīng) for over 20 years. Although the external forms changed, the Taijiquan (功夫 gōng fu) he studied and modified is now the most popular style of Taijiquan, known as the big frame (大架式 dà jiàshì) of Yang Family Taijiquan (楊氏太極拳 yáng shì tài jí quán).

Afterwards, Wu Jian Quan's (吳鑑泉 wú jiàn quán) Wu Family Taijiquan (吳氏太極拳 wú shì tài jí quán), Wu Yu Xiang's (武禹襄 wǔ yǔ xiāng) Wu Family Taijiquan (武氏太極拳 wǔ shì tàijíquán), and Sun Lu Tang's (孫綠堂 sūn lù táng) Sun Family Taijiquan (孫氏太極拳 sūn shì tài jí quán) followed. Although their external forms differ, they are all officially recognized as Taijiquan. This is because the internal disciplines are the same in all styles of Taijiquan, despite the variations in form.

In order to make the 25 key disciplines accessible, I created 4 sections with my teacher's help. The first section describes the Law of Body (身法 shēnfǎ), the second section details the Law of Mind (心法 xīnfǎ), the third section addresses the Law of Reeling Silk (纏絲法 chán sī fǎ), and the fourth section presents the 4 major characteristics (四大特點 sì dà tè diǎn).

The heritage of Chen Family Taijiquan started from the first ancestor (始祖 shǐzǔ) of the Chen family, Chen Bu (陳卜 chén bǔ), a pioneer, who in 1372 settled down in Chen Village. Taijiquan as a complete system was realized by a 9th generation family member named Chen Wang Ting (陳王廷 chén wáng tíng: 1600 - 1680). It has been transmitted and further developed by the Chen family since then. Each of the key disciplines manifest differently, depending on a practitioner's level of study. Practitioners are able to measure and understand their current levels based on the standards of the key disciplines. Unfortunately, without having a solid grasp of the key disciplines of Taijiquan, practice can be likened to meaningless motions.

What is 'Fang Song'?

Before I explain the key disciplines, it is crucial to understand the meaning of the word '放鬆 fàng sōng'.

The dictionary's definition is 'to put 放 Fàng' and 'pine tree 鬆 sōng'. The direct translation is 'to put a pine tree'. Before discussing Fang Song, it is necessary to savor the taste and meaning of the pine tree '鬆 sōng'.

'Song' is now used as pine tree 'sōng 松' in the simplified Chinese (简體 jiǎn tǐ). However in traditional Chinese (繁體 fán tǐ), it is used with 'biāo 髟' which means a pine tree or a mop of hair (bushy hair)- 'song 鬆'. It describes a shape like the top of a pine tree. When looking at a pine tree, we can see there is a root that exists underneath the ground, a trunk that lives above it, with branches and leaves that sprout from the stem. This is the true meaning of 'song'.

In other words, when practicing 'fang song' in Taijiquan, the legs should be as solid as the root, the body should be as upright as the trunk, and the arms, neck and head should be loose like the branches and leaves on a pine tree.

In general, it is often said 'efface power or remove force' when using the term 'Fang Song', but this is a misunderstanding (曲解 qū jiě). It is more appropriate to use expressions such as 'be soft' or 'loosen up the stiffness (硬直 yìng zhí) of the body'. This more accurately describes Fang Song versus 'efface power or remove force'. How could one grab an object or even stand without some force? Being soft and loosening up means to softly relax while allowing minimal force by releasing tension. For instance, when practicing Taijiquan straight sword, the sword would fly out of one's hands if there was no force utilized. Minimal force is required to grab the sword, however the body must remain loose to attain softness and expand when practicing with this weapon with the correct 'fang song'. When reaching the true status of '鬆 sōng', every single joint, muscle, bone experiences a feeling of great expansion and extension. This is the true concept and meaning of 'song'.

Also, a pine tree is one of the ten traditional symbols of longevity; it implies youth and unyielding spirit. This meaning is similarly used in Chen Family Taijiquan. When practicing, the concept of Fang Song should always be adhered to and requires a detached temperament (氣像 qì xiàng). The true meaning of 'fang song' is that 'fang' indicates to 'fully put down'. So it is liberally translated: 'fully put down a pine tree'. In practical translation, it is to deeply relax the mind and body as if 'dropping' a pine tree into the ground. The message is to lay down the body and mind, be soft and open, loosen up and expand, in order to attain a state of deep relaxation (弛緩 chí huǎn).

Metaphorically speaking, 'fang song' in Chen Family Taijiquan refers to the body and mind; the whole body resembles the external form of a pine tree. The legs, like the solid root of the tree, the torso like the trunk, and the arms like the widely spread-open branches. The mind should be like a shadow beneath the pine tree, covering it in silence and calmness. The pine tree, with superior 'fang song', would have a large frame casting a big shadow, whereas the pine tree with inferior 'fang song' would possess a slighter frame and therefore produce a smaller shadow. In approaching the ultimate zenith (極致 jízhì) of 'song', it is possible to learn deeply and profoundly understand the foundation of true salient power (勁力 jìn lì) known as 'ward-off' (掤勁 pēng jìn). Without the understanding of 'fang song', it is impossible to start or complete Taijiquan practice.

The Law of the Body (身法 shēn fǎ)

Through the Law of Body, the principle of the negative and the positive (陰陽原理 yīn yáng yuán lǐ) is understood and manifests in the body.

1. 虛領頂勁 Xū Lǐng Dǐng Jìn

Meaning (意味 yì wèi)

Xu: Empty   **Ling:** Make   **Ding:** crown/top of the head   **Jin:** upright or solid

Direct translation (直譯 zhí yì)

Make the crown of the head empty and upright.

Practical translation (意譯 yì yì)

Deeply relax the neck so it is very soft.

Lift up the crown of the head toward the sky solidly.

Annotation (注解 zhù jiě)

This is to open the center of the crown of the head (百會穴 bǎi huì xué) while softening the neck (cervical). Its purpose is to deeply relax (fang song) the neck and head. Tuck in the chin slightly in order to stretch out the back of the neck upwards. The whole head should feel like it is dangling in the air. This spontaneously opens the cranium and cervical 1 (atlas), while a suspended feeling from the crown is experienced. A practitioner who suffers from stiffness and/or herniated disks of the neck can benefit greatly by practicing this discipline (要訣 yào jué).

By practicing 'xu ling ding jin', both the meridian point 'bai hui' and the Atlas cervical open and become supple, which will maximize vitalization of the pineal gland. This is a very important key unlocking the first gate that leads to the 25 key disciplines of Chen Family Taijiquan.

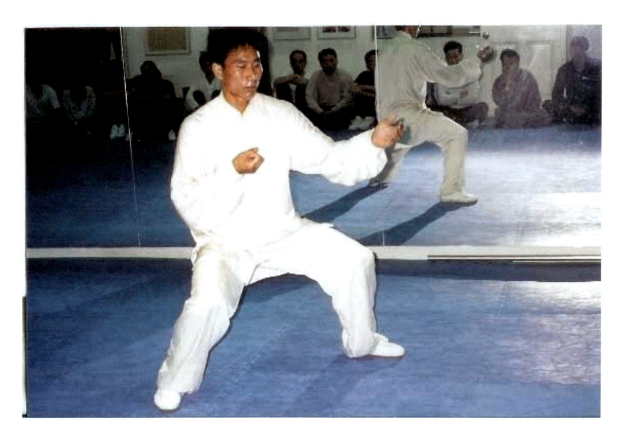

Master Chen Bing in May 2000 - Seoul, South Korea

This was my first encounter with my Taiji teacher Chen Bing. In 2000, he made his first foreign trip to South Korea to promote the original Taijiquan. After his appearance and knowledgeable lectures, the standard of Taijiquan was entirely changed in Korea.

2. 鬆肩沈肘 Sōng Jiān Chěn Zhǒu

Meaning

Song: Loosen up, decompress tension or relax

Jian: Shoulder   **Chen:** Sink or immerse   **Zhou:** Elbow

Direct translation

Loosen up the shoulder and immerge the elbow.

Practical translation

Softly open the shoulder joint (關節 guān jié) to relax and sink down the elbow in order to relax the wrist and fingertips.

Annotation

Compared to other key disciplines, this principle is relatively easier to learn than others. However, it is not possible to deepen the meaning of it if a previous discipline, 'xu ling ding jin', is not preceded. If the shoulders are relaxed, they feel as if they are lengthening the shoulder joint horizontally. The entire arm becomes very heavy when the elbow is lowered, followed by the wrist. The palm should be naturally opened; it possesses the meridian point 'the palace of toil' (勞宮穴 láo gōng xué) which is at the center of the palm. All ten fingers should be spaced naturally, unclosed and without tension.

If 'song jian chen zhou' is complete, the shoulder joint opens wide, the elbow gets heavy and the palm and fingers experience a sensation of swelling. If a practitioner has an injury, or is unable to raise their arms, it is acceptable to practice without raising the arms, or, to slightly raise them under the instruction of qualified teachers. Generally, it tends to bring physical discomfort or stiffness of the arms when opening a rigid arms' joint by relaxation (song) to achieve relaxation.

Through the key discipline of 'song jian chen zhou', the thoracic area will enjoy better conditions to relax and expand more deeply. With both arms raised, it is called standing post (站庄 zhàn zhuāng); without raising the arms, it is called calm mind practice (靜心功 jìng xīn gōng).

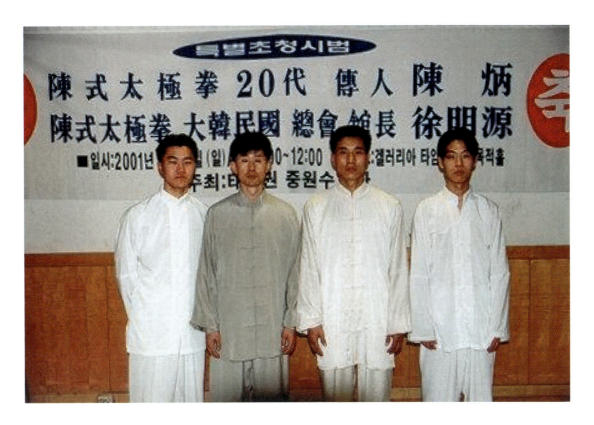

Chen Family Taijiquan demonstration in Daejeon, South Korea

on January 14 2001

From left, Hans Oh (the first foreign disciple of Grand Master Chen Yu), Myeongwon Seo (the first foreign disciple of Grand Master Chen Xiaoxing), Master Chen Bing, Bosco Baek (senior disciple of Master Chen Bing)

Korean disciples of the Chen family were produced by Master Chen Bing's contribution and influence.

3. 含胸塌腰 Hán Xiōng Tā Yāo

Meaning

Han: Incubate   **Xiong:** Chest   **Ta:** Suspend   **Yao:** Lower back

Direct translation

Incubate the chest and suspend the lower back.

Practical translation

Hollow the chest as if carefully holding an infant, soften the lower back and relax the spine downwards without any tension.

尾閭中正 Wěi Lú Zhōng Zhèng

Meaning

Wei: Tail   **Lu:** Town or door in the corner of town

Zhong: Center   **Zheng:** Upright

Direct translation

The door of the tail is centered and upright.

Practical translation

Position the tailbone in the center, lower it down and keep it upright.

<u>Annotation</u>

The key principles of 'han xiong ta yao' and 'wei lu zhong zheng' are the most important key disciplines in Chen Family Taijiquan because they are hard to learn and require the delicate and hands-on corrections of a teacher. In general, most instructors and practitioners overdo it, by overtly caving in the upper chest, which actually creates stiffness in the body. The true 'han xiong' is not visible because it is sensed internally. The reason is that the full depth of relaxation cannot be seen with the naked eye, but rather, practitioners first learn it physically and then must experience it deeply in a state of internal observation (內觀 nèi guān).

In Chinese medicine, the chest area is considered one of 'the three chests (三焦 sān jiāo)' which includes the upper chest (上焦 shàng jiāo), the middle chest (中焦 zhōngjiāo), and the lower chest (下焦 xià jiāo). The upper chest is located above the diaphragm (heart and lungs), the middle chest is located from the diaphragm to the navel (spleen, stomach and liver), and the lower chest is located below the navel (kidney, large intestine, small intestine and bladder).

'Han xiong' is to control 'the upper chest'. As the heart is the motor of blood circulation, which is directly related to emotions, it should be treated carefully – like caring for a baby. Therefore, relax the chest as carefully as cradling and soothing an infant.

In addition, if the previous keys 'xu ling ding jin' and 'song jian chen zhou' are executed properly, a student is able to genuinely understand 'hollowing the chest' (han xiong) and reach 'suspending the lower back' (ta yao), a state in which the erector spinae (脊椎起立筋 jǐ zhuī qǐ lì jīn) of the lower back possesses no curve (concave or convex) and is free of any tension.

When reaching 'ta yao', the tailbone (coccyx) relaxes spontaneously, is suspended and dangles downward. It feels like a plum dangling or dropping. With this key, secret discipline, Chen Family Taijiquan practitioners can fully fill and expand (擴張 kuò zhāng) the thoracic (upper and middle back), lumbar (lower back), and coccyx (tailbone). Many of the descendants in the Chen Family Taijiquan lineage do not suffer from lower back pain, or herniated discs as a result of mastering this **'top secret'** (極祕 jí mì) discipline. 'Spine back relax combine' (脊背鬆合 jǐ bèi sōng hé), which is one of Master Chen Bing's unique Taiji relaxation practices, is the most effective way to grasp the secret to this principle.

If 'han xiong ta yao' and 'wei lu zhong zheng' are fully realized, the 'elixir field' (丹田 dāntián) and 'life door' (命門 mìngmén) that is located between lumbar 2 and 3 on the back will horizontally face one another. This is the opening condition of the girdle penetration vessel that is one of 'eight extraordinary vessels' (奇經八脈 qí jīng bā mài). With 'xu ling ding jin', the center of crown and perineum (會陰穴 huì yīn xué) interpenetrates energy (qi) vertically throughout the spine.

In other words, 'the girdle penetration vessel' (帶脈 dài mài) and the 'interpenetration vessel through the spine' (衝脈 chōng mài) will flow through naturally. Mastering 'han xiong ta yao' and 'wei lu zhong zheng' is the start of authentic Taijiquan practice.

After becoming very proficient in 'xu ling ding jin', 'song jian chen zhou', 'han xiong ta yao' and 'wei lu zhong zheng', expanding and relaxing the entire spine is achievable. 'Xu ling ding Jin' deals with the cranium (head) and the cervical (neck), 'song jian chen zhou' addresses the shoulders and arms, 'han xiong ta yao' focuses on the chest, thoracic (back) and lumbar (lower back), while 'wei lu zhong zheng' is concerned with the sacrum and coccyx (tailbone) relaxing and expanding. If they are all well executed, it is as if one thread is stretched up and down (上下 shàng xià), from the neck to tailbone. It feels like the top of one's head is rising up to the sky, while the back, lower back and tailbone drop/sink downwards.

This is the crowning gem (白眉 bái méi) of Chen Family Taijiquan, and causes 'expansion of the spine' (脊椎擴張 jǐ zhuī kuò zhāng). When it is mastered, every joint in the spine is maximized to expand and get refreshed. In fact, I even created a definition for this one as 'spine refreshment' (脊椎回復生氣 jǐ zhuī huí fù shēng qì). While avoiding spinal injuries, the direct descendants of the oldest lineage, genuine Chen Family Taijiquan practitioners, have found the secret to anti-aging by mastering these key disciplines.

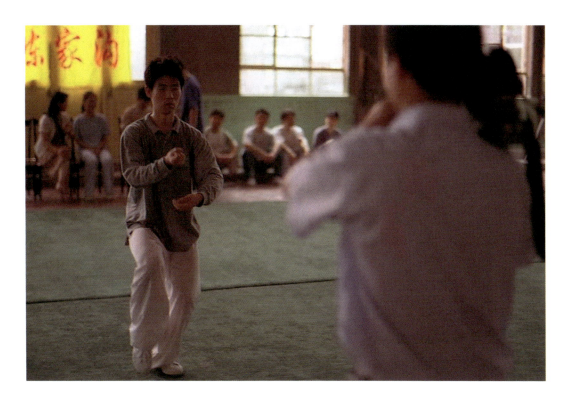

My first Chenjiagou visit in August 2002

After becoming a national champion of Taijiquan in Korea in 2002, I was invited to demonstrate Taijiquan in Chenjiagou.

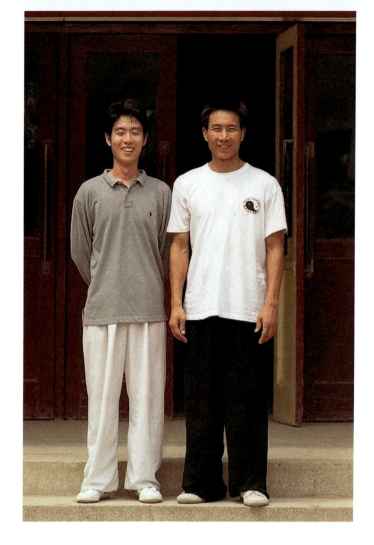

My wonderful Taiji teacher Chen Bing and I

Chenjiagou - August 2002

Personally, I was very moved by his personality even more than his amazing Taijiquan skills.

4. 屈膝鬆胯 Qū Xī Sōng Kuà

Meaning

Qu: Bend   **Xi:** Knee   **Song:** Relax   **Kua:** Hip/ groin/ inguinal crease

Direct translation

Bend the knees and relax the hip.

Practical translation

Relax the hip by bending the knees.

Annotation

If the previous disciplines aim to take control of the whole spine in the upper body, this key discipline governs the hips and legs in the lower body. While bending both knees slightly, one is able to fold the hips backwards in to the body creating a space to relax the hip joint (胯 kuà). In order to trigger the 4 extraordinary vessels (yang-heel, yang-linking, yin-heel and yin-linking) of the 8 extraordinary vessels in the lower body naturally, the weight of the body should be on the heel of the foot instead of the toes; and the knee can't hang over beyond the toes. Two thirds of the weight goes on the heel and one third of the weight goes on the front part of the foot. From the side view, the ankle, hip, shoulder and ear must maintain a vertical alignment to achieve a correct posture.

By 'qu xi song kua', the upper body becomes the emptiness of yin (陰虛 yīn xū) and, at the same time, the lower body becomes the fullness of yang (陽實 yáng shí). Due to a characteristic of yin (the negative) and yang (the positive), the yin energy (陰氣 yīn qì) in the upper body is lowered (下降 xià jiàng) down and the yang energy '陽氣 yáng qì' in the lower body is raised (上昇 shàngshēng). That is to say the energies of the upper and lower body will be combined in the elixir field (丹田 dān tián) which, by the principle of 'qu xi song kua', is the connector between the upper and lower body. This is called the formation of the elixir field (丹田形成 dān tián xíng chéng). It can't be called Taijiquan if one of the knees is straightened or not bent because it violates this principle.

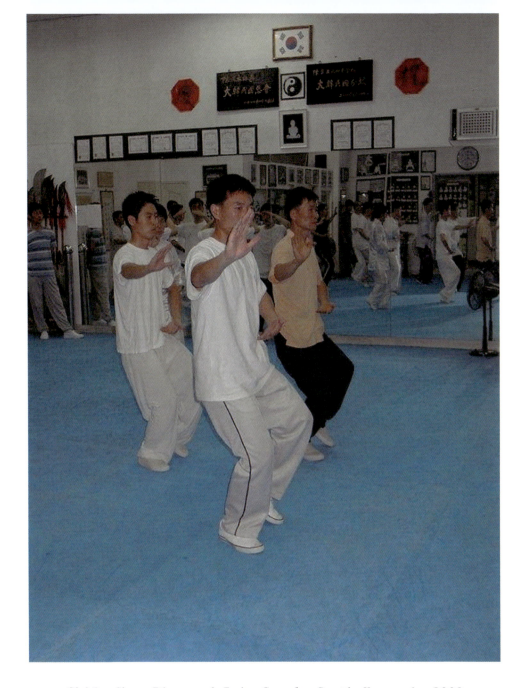

Shifu Chen Bing and I in Seoul, South Korea in 2003

This picture was taken right before I moved to the United States of America in 2003.

5. 垂臀圓襠 Chuí Tún Yuán Dāng

Meaning

Chui: Hang or dangle **Tun:** Buttocks

Yuan: Round or circle **Dang:** Groin or crotch

Direct translation

Hang the buttocks and round the groin.

Practical translation

Relax the buttock muscle, dangle the tailbone and round the crotch.

Annotation

The buttocks should be relaxed and loosened to hang down. It's shape should be round. The groin (inner thigh) should be circular. The meaning of 'chui tun' signifies that the tailbone is dropped down by relaxing the buttocks muscles. In human anatomy, the tailbone (coccyx) itself is already rolled-up. Therefore, it can't achieve the status of relaxation (fang song) due to tension around the lower back and abdomen, especially if there is an artificial effort to tuck-in or roll it up in a constrained manner.

The concept of 'yuan dang' is not just about making an arch shape with the legs. It involves the arches of the feet and knees facing vertically, while the groin opens into an ellipse (椭圆 tuǒ yuán). If the buttocks remain relaxed, the tailbone will gently dangle down, allowing the thighs to open unaffectedly. This is true 'yuan dang'.

Any exaggerated effort to open the thigh, knee, or an attempt to produce a full circle with the legs does not necessarily qualify as 'yuan dang'. If 'chui tun yuan dang' is realized, it will create elasticity in the entire lower body. This is called the root of the legs (脚根 jiǎo gēn) or the root of dantian (丹田根 dān tián gēn). In addition, the hips or knees should not be collapsed or broken when discharging force or performing push-hands (推手 tuī shǒu).

The third discipline in the law of body 'relax the chest and lower back - han xiong ta yao, position the tailbone in the center, lower it down and keep it upright - wei lu zhong zheng' should be maintained along with the fifth discipline (relax the buttocks and round the legs - chui tun yuan dang) and sixth discipline (maintain the central status -li shen zhong zheng) as the basic foundation at all times.

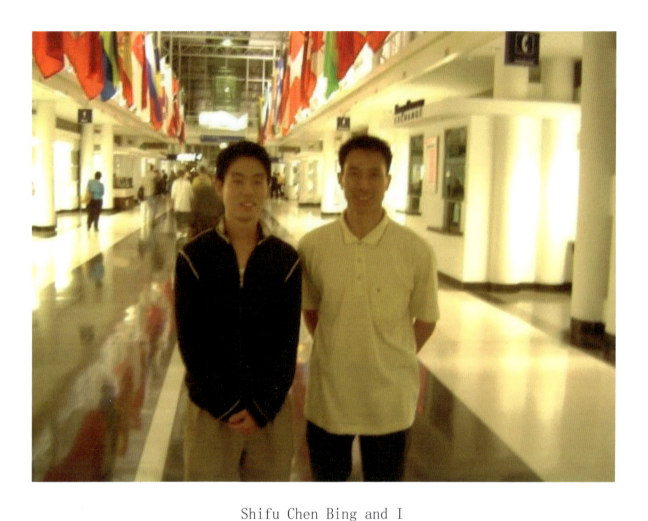

Shifu Chen Bing and I

Chicago O' Hare International Airport on September 9, 2004

I am the first person who brought my Shifu to Chicago on September 2004 and started sending him to various locations in the USA. From this year onwards, Master Chen started gaining international fame as a great Taijiquan teacher.

6. 下盘稳固 Xià Pán Wěn Gù

Meaning

Xia: Under   **Pan**: Tray or base   **Wen**: Comfortable   **Gu**: Solid

Direct translation

Be comfortable and solid under a tray.

Practical translation

The legs (lower body) become comfortable and solid as a root.

Annotation

When training Taijiquan, the lower body should be rooted into the ground, which is sturdy and solid. As a tree with a weak root can't sprout a healthy stem or leaf, the lower body should be like a solid root while the thigh and knee should be fixed absolutely. Practitioners are able to build up a strong lower body through a lot of time and practice. The stronger the lower body gets in Taijiquan, the stronger the torso and arms will get as well. As jumping depends on how much one bends their legs, an elasticity(弹性 tán xìng) like a spring will be produced when 'xia pan wen gu' is enabled. It can be said that one is able to produce more power in the upper body if one has developed the power in the lower body. If a senior citizen or physically challenged individual practices, it is recommended to run a parallel course combining 'Taiji Relaxation Practice' (fang song gong which is the unique style of Master Chen Bing's) and 'Reeling Silk Practice' to increase their practice time but be careful not to over train. A practitioner is able to calibrate the time and amount of practice based on their skill level.

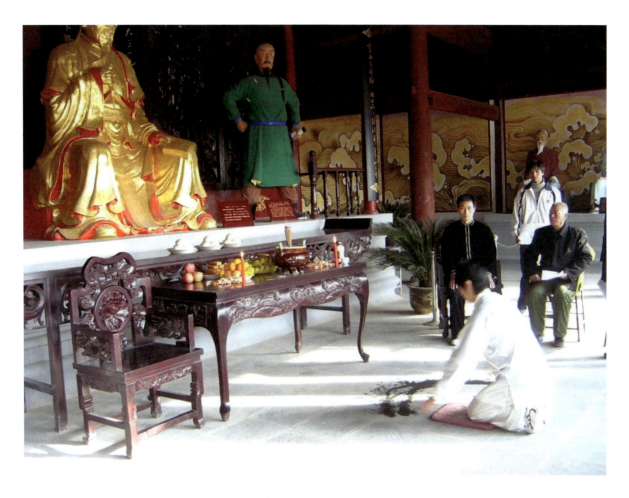

My disciple ceremony on Christmas day of 2005 in Chenjiagou

My disciple ceremony was small and very intimate, and was one of the most unforgettable experiences in my life.

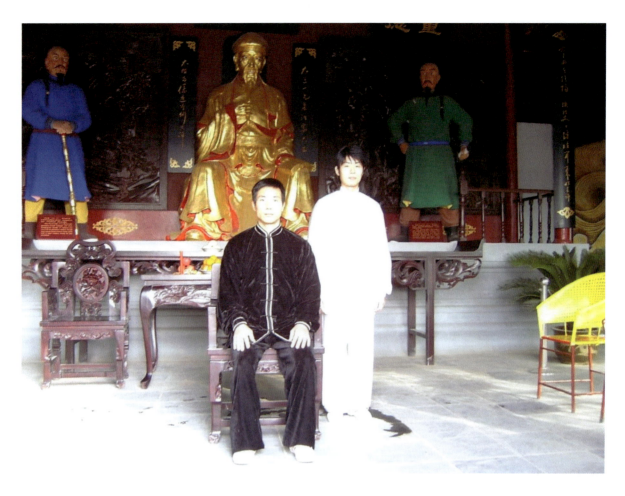

Shifu Chen Bing and I on Christmas day of 2005 in Chenjiagou

On December 25 2005, I became a formal disciple as a 13th successor of Chen Family Taijiquan.

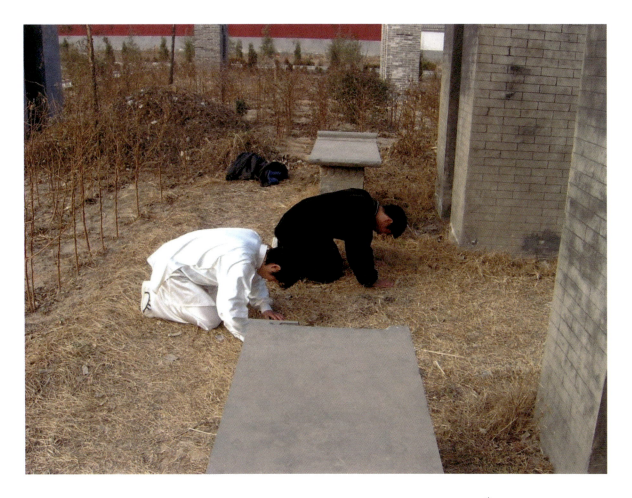

Shifu Chen Bing and I bowing to the tombstone of the 17th generation representative of the Chen family, Chen Fake, after my disciple ceremony

Shifu Chen Bing asked me to go to the graveyard of his ancestors after the disciple ceremony. We both bowed to each ancestor's grave to greet a discipleship and life time pledge to carry the family art of Taijiquan.

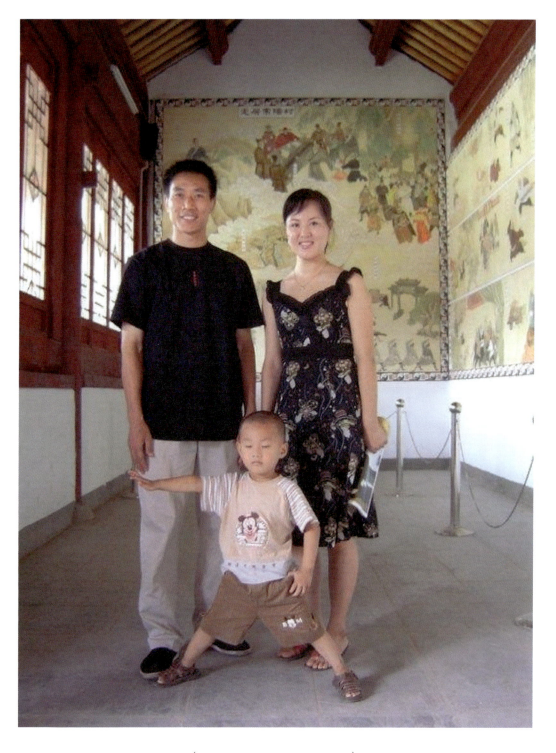

Shifu Chen Bing, his wife (Shimu Li Shuang Ling) and his son Chen Shaotong

August 2005 in Chenjiagou at the Chen Family Taiji Museum

7. 身中正 Lì Shēn Zhōng Zhèng

Meaning

Li: Stand up   **Shen:** Body   **Zhong:** Center or important   **Zheng:** Correct, accurate or rightly

Direct translation

The body stands up in the center correctly.

Practical translation

The body's posture and positioning should be visibly upright and straight in all directions.

Annotation

Positioning the body in the center line means there is an upright (no leaning) posture when looking at one's self from the front, side and back, no matter the angle.

This can be simply defined as central status in English and there are 2 types. The first type is called an upright central status (正的中正 zhèng de zhōng zhèng) and the second is called a leaning (diagonal) central status (斜的中正 xié de zhōng zhèng).

The most effective way to learn the upright central equilibrium status is to perform the 'calm mind practice' (靜心功 jìng xīn gōng) and 'standing post' (站庄 zhàn zhuāng). In terms of self-correction for 'li shen zhong zheng', vertically align the ear, shoulder, hip and ankle bone via your side profile. This is a general description of the first type of central status (central equilibrium) condition. The second type of central status might not be easy to comprehend without understanding the first kind of central status. While maintaining the ideal straight alignment of the 4 points that are the ear, shoulder, hip and ankle, leaning forward or backward is possible depending on forms, combat situations and martial applications. For example, the Old Frame form has a posture called 'oblique walk' (斜行 xié xíng) which involves a lean forward, requiring the second type of leaning central status. Another example of this second type of central status is a posture called 'white ape offers fruit (白猿獻果 bái yuán xiàn guǒ)' which requires backward-leaning in Chen Taiji straight sword. The main purpose of these leaning postures is to internally feel the formation of the elixir field which has heaviness, fullness and openness while leaning. As the Taiji diagram displays, any changes or fluctuations are able to occur if the key principles are actively in place.

In fact, 'li shen zhong zheng' is not feasible without the preparation provided by the six key disciplines that precede it. This rule should be maintained at all times, not only when in a stationary position, but also when moving the body (advancing, retreating, and stepping sideways). If the body does not obey these 2 types of central statuses, it is not true 'li shen zhong zheng'.

'Li shen zhong zheng's 'zhong' means the center, but it means 'important' as well. This is a double entendre of Chinese literature (中文 zhōngwén).

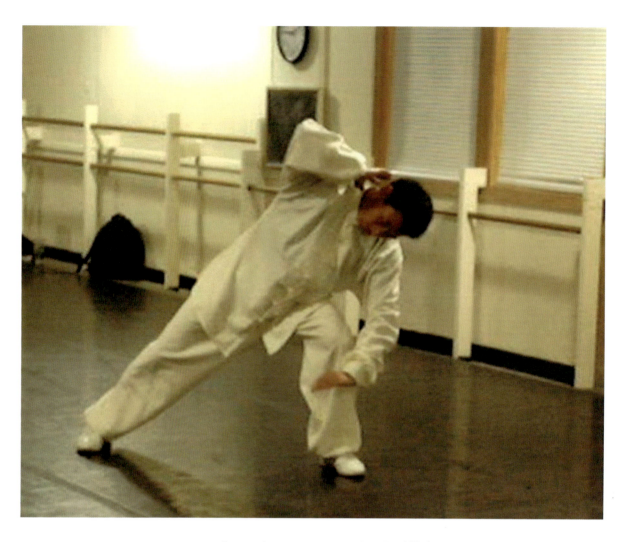

Shifu Chen Bing's 'Oblique Walking' (斜行 xiéxíng)

in Old Frame First Road – April 2008 in Chicago

This is a good example of the second type of leaning central status.

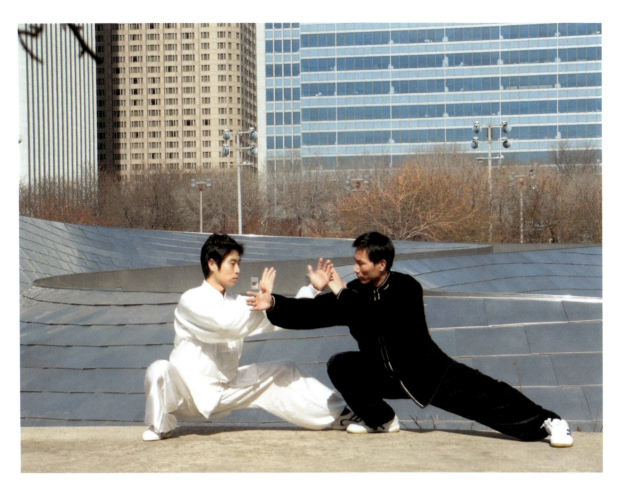

Shifu Chen Bing and I performing

'Big Roll-back' (大履推手 dà lǚ tuī shǒu)

May 2006 in Chicago

8. 上虛下實 Shàng Xū Xià Shí

Meaning

Shang: Upper **Xu:** Empty or not be **Xia:** Lower **Shi:** (Fully) full or fill

Direct translation

The upper is empty and the lower is full.

Practical translation

The upper body becomes the negative and the lower body becomes the positive.

虛實分明 Xū Shí Fēn Míng

Meaning

Xu: Empty **Shi:** (Fully) full or fill **Fen:** Split or separate **Ming:** Clear

Direct translation

The empty and the full are clearly split.

Practical translation

The negative (emptiness and lightness) and the positive (fullness and heaviness) should be split and separated clearly.

Annotation

The human body can be divided into two sections which are the upper and lower body. 'Shang xu xia shi' describes when the upper body becomes as light as emptiness while the lower body becomes solid as fullness. In the theory of yin and yang, being empty is the negative (陰 yīn) and being full is the positive (陽 yáng). When the upper body reaches a negative state, the energy of the upper body will sink downward into the elixir field. Conversely, when the lower body attains a positive state, the energy of the lower body will rise upward into the elixir field. This is how the core of the elixir field is formed when the negative and positive reach their peak. The characteristics of the negative, some of which are female, lowering, closing, soft, slow, sleeping, and the moon can create the birth of life. This is why Taiji practitioners strive for making the upper body as negative.

If the upper becomes 1 pound and the lower becomes 5 pounds, this condition is thought of as a stable and healthy condition. If reversed, it would be totally opposite.

'Xu shi fen ming' implies the condition that one of the legs becomes the negative (虛 xū) while the other leg becomes the positive (實 shí) - just as one of the arms becomes the positive while the other arm becomes the negative. For instance, while executing the posture of 'Lazy about tying the coat (懶扎衣 lǎn zhá yī), the right leg becomes the positive (fullness) as the left leg becomes the negative (emptiness); the right arm becomes the positive as the left arm becomes the negative.

Another meaning of 'xu shi fen ming' is 'rise lower open close' (昇降開合 shēng jiàng kāi hé). 'Lowering and closing' is a characteristic of the negative and 'rising and opening' is a characteristic of the positive. At all times, expressions of the negative and the positive must be separated clearly when practicing Taijiquan.

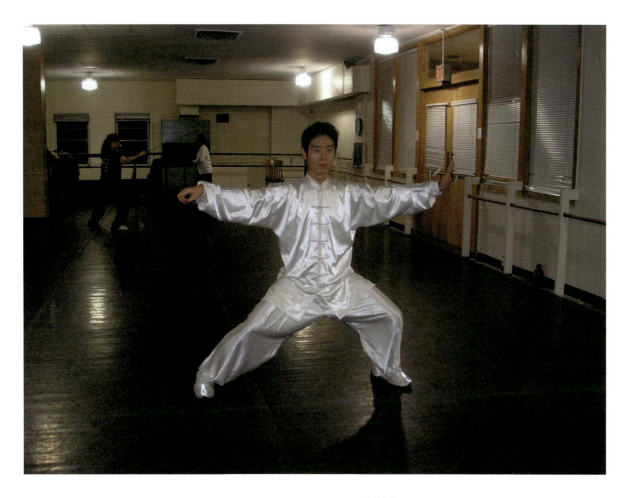

Me performing 'Single Whip' (單鞭 dān biān)

November 2008 - Chicago, IL

9. 八面支撑 Bā Miàn Zhī Chēng

Meaning

Ba: Eight   **Mian:** Direction or side   **Zhi:** Support or sustain   **Cheng:** Endure or hold up

Direct translation

Supporting eight sides.

Practical translation

There is an elasticity to support from all directions.

Annotation

The eight sides are East, West, North and South as the 4 main directions (cardinal: 四正點 sì zhèng diǎn), with North-East, North-West, South-East and South-West as the 4 supportive directions (intercardinal: 四隅點 sì yú diǎn). In the practices of Chen Family Taijiquan, all postures should be adaptable and 'nimble-lively' (活 ling huó) to be able to change in all eight directions. It does not just mean directions, but actually, it is also required to understand what is called 'ward-off' through the postures.

There are two meanings of 'ward-off' (掤勁 péng jìn). The first one is inner elasticity, like a bowstring, and the second one is an application to extrude an opponent away from, or off the body. If the previous 8 disciplines are fulfilled, the front, back, and side of the foot produces natural elasticity and resilience from the bottom. Whereas the upper body is relaxed, it experiences a state of softness and being fully expanded. This is true 'elastic support in all directions'. It should be maintained at all times while training, especially during reeling silk practice (纏絲功 chán sī gōng), forms (套路 tào lù) and the 5 kinds of push-hands.

There are eight forces of Taijiquan, which are ward-off (掤 péng), roll-back (捋 lǔ), press (擠 jǐ), push (按 àn), pull-down (採 cǎi), split (挒 liè), elbow stroke (肘 zhǒu) and shoulder stroke (靠 kào). When the true inner expansion inside the body is realized, ward off becomes the mother force to supports the changes to roll-back, press, push, pull-down, split, elbow stroke and shoulder stroke.

When practicing the standing post, the 9 key disciplines must be gently in place, with all of one's heart involved. The same key disciplines should be applied in the practice of reeling silk or forms as the basic requirements.

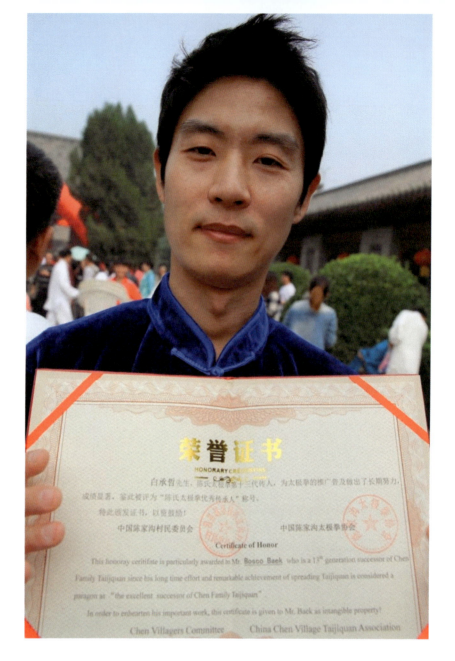

I was appointed as the

'Chenjiagou Intangible Cultural Chen Family Taijiquan Excellent Successor'

(陈家沟非物质文化陈氏太极拳优秀传承人)

by the Chen Villagers Committee and China Chen Village Taijiquan

Association on October 5 2014 in Chenjiagou

The Law of the Mind (心法 Xīn Fǎ)

If the Laws of the Body have been fulfilled (先行 xiānxíng), then it is possible to practice the Law of the Mind.

The Law of the Mind is at the core of how Chen Family Taijquan becomes an internal practice (內家拳 nèi jiā quán).

10. 全身放鬆 Quán Shēn Fàng Sōng

Meaning

Quan: Whole   **Shen:** Body   **Fang:** Put   **Song:** Relax

Direct translation

Relax the whole body deeply.

Practical translation

Relax the whole body evenly so that every part is very soft.

Annotation

It is easy to say 'relax' in words, but it is not easy in practice. In order to relax the entire body, there is a specific order to undergo, from head to toe. First of all, envision a white board. Draw every body part on the board and try to sense it.

Basic 'fang song' (whole body relaxation) order is as follows:

1. Head

2. Neck

3. Shoulders

4. Arms

5. Chest

6. Waist

7. Legs

8. Feet

With eyes closed and using your mind, slowly feel, be aware of the body and try to relax. After getting familiar with the basic Fang Song order, practice it in detail.

Here is a detailed relaxation (fang song) order:

1. Top of head (bai hui)

2. Forehead

3. Eye brow

4. The center of eye brow - 3rd eye or upper elixir field (上丹田 shàng dān tián)

5. Nose

6. Tip of nose

7. Lips

8. Teeth

9. Back of neck

10. Front of neck

11. Left of neck

12. Right of neck

13. Shoulders

14. Elbows

15. Wrist

16. Palms

17. Fingers

18. Fingertips

19. Upper chest: middle elixir field (中丹田 zhōng dān tián)

20. Upper back

21. Middle of the back (solar plexus)

22. Lower abdomen: lower elixir field (下丹田 xià dān tián)

23. Lower back

24. Hips

25. Buttocks

26. Thighs

27. Back of thighs (hamstring)

28. Knees

29. Shins

30. Calves

31. Ankles

32. Heels

33. Arches of the feet

34. Soles

35. Toes

36. End of toes

Use intention (thought, 意念 yì niàn) and follow slowly in this order. Then the mind (心 xīn) becomes comfortable and reaches a state of deep relaxation. The Law of Intention and the Law of the Mind are different. The mind is the master of intention (thought/meaning). When speaking of intention (意 yì) in Chinese, what is meant is that intention is a sound (音 yīn) made by the mind (心 xīn). In general, it is often expressed as 'empty mind', however this is incorrect. The mind cannot be empty. For instance, we dream while sleeping. Dreaming is an action of mind stemming from various stimuli and emotions that move the mind while awake. So a 'dream' is a medium influenced by such factors. The mind is an active thing which works briskly, 24 hours a day. In other words, it can't be empty!

Even if the mind cannot be empty, it is possible to calm it by using intention (意 yì). If there are distracting or worldly thoughts (雜念 zá niàn) while practicing this 'whole body relaxation', then just watch them. Those distracting thoughts are part of the mind's action. They only multiply and intensify when we try to block them out.

Acquaint yourself slowly with the orders of 'whole body relaxation' and practice. One may attain a very deep sense of relaxation rather easily. For example, one could feel that the 25-minute standing post or calming mind practice goes by too fast, feeling like a 5-minute practice after a few months. This is already a great achievement and clear evidence that a practitioner of this ilk is able to rest the mind by practicing the intention to attain true relaxation, as well as the experience of 'fang song'. Otherwise, the standing post would be a most boring exercise that many students try to avoid practicing unless having adequate comprehension. The order of 'fang song' is flexible and can change under a teacher's instruction afterwards. For example, internal organs (the five viscera and the six entrails) are added at the practitioner's discretion depending on their level of study.

For instance, it is feasible to perform it in the following sequences:

1. Bladder
2. Liver
3. Heart
4. Stomach

5. Lung

6. Kidney

It could be from the left to the right, from right to left, or even from bottom to top.

The discipline of 'Quan Shen Fang Song' is the most crucial within the Law of the Mind. Regardless of physical strength, capability or age, one can practice this by lying down on the floor.

When true relaxation happens, three parts of the body become very heavy. They are arms, dantian and legs. They are called 3 heavinesses (三重 sān zhòng) that have to be maintained all times while training Taijiquan. The flesh of a human is limited (有限 yǒu xiàn), yet the mind is unlimited (無限 wú xiàn). The term 'fang song' is not the limited meaning. For instance, you may fang song the skin, pores, ligaments, tendons and specific body parts that are injured. In fact, 'fang song' has no limit in application.

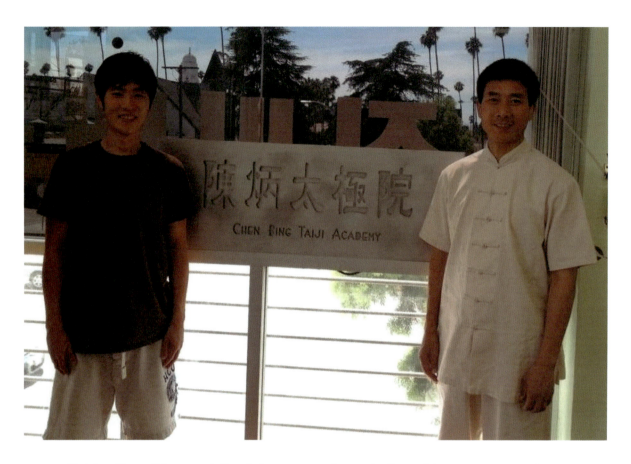

Shifu Chen Bing and I with a new sign of Chen Bing Taiji Academy made by Pamela Hom in May 2012 - Los Angeles, CA

11. 心氣下降 Xīn Qì Xià Jiàng

Meaning

Xin: Mind   **Qi**: Energy   **Xia**: Down or low   **Jiang**: Go down

Direct translation

Go down the energy of mind to the low.

Practical translation

Stabilize the mind and make it comfortable to harness the 'fire of the mind' (心火 xīn huǒ).

Annotation

In this discipline, there are five intents. The first is not to be anxious (不急躁 bù jí zào), the second is to be stable (安静 ān jìng), the third is to ease the heart (放心 fàng xīn), the fourth is to feel easy (舒心 shū xīn), and the fifth is to be tranquil (平心 píng xīn). With the combination of these five, the fire of the mind (心火 xīn huǒ) spontaneously goes down (下降 xià jiàng) to help vitalize the water energy of the kidneys (腎水 shèn shuǐ).

If one understands 'yin and yang', then the five elements can be understood as well. A characteristic of 'yin' (the negative) is cold, so it is with the element of 'water'. Conversely, a characteristic of 'yang' (the positive) is heat, therefore it is associated with 'fire'. Water always falls from top to bottom whereas fire consistently rises from the bottom to the top. Therefore, the heart, which is independently located from other internal organs is considered to have the characteristic of 'fire', while the kidneys, which are the internal organs located lower than the rest, are considered to be of 'water'.

In the yin-yang and five elements, the heart (心臟 xīn zàng) is fire (火 huǒ), the kidney (腎臟 shèn zàng) is water (水 shuǐ), the liver is wood (木 mù), the lungs are metal or stone (jīn), and the spleen is ground earth (土 tǔ). The five elements always change for coexistence (相生 xiāng shēng) and incompatibility (相剋 xiāng kè).

The coexistence is to nurture and produce harmony. A tree grows if there is plenty of water (water produces tree, 水生木 shuǐ shēng mù); fire works well if there are plenty of trees (wood produces fire, 木生火 mù shēng huǒ); Earth is formed as fire turns everything to ash (fire produces Earth, 火生土 huǒ shēng tǔ); Earth produces stone after becoming rigid (ground produces stone, 土生 tǔ shēng jīn); stone accumulates morning dew after a night, or hot metal from a smithy needs water to cool (stone or metal produces water, 生水 jīn shēng shuǐ).

On the other hand, the incompatibility is to contradict each other. Fire cannot burn off stone (fire conflicts with stone, 火剋 huǒ kè jīn), a tree is unable to grow in stone or metal (metal and stone conflicts with a tree, 剋木 jīn kè mù); ground space is lacking if there are too many trees (tree conflicts with ground, 木剋土 mù kè tǔ); water is insufficient if there is a lot of ground (earth conflicts with water, 土剋水 tǔ kè shuǐ) and water extinguishes fire (water conflicts with fire, 水剋火 shuǐ kè huǒ).

In the five elements, fire should be lowered because the heart is thought of as fire (火 huǒ). Sinking the energy (氣 qì) down to the bottom helps maximize the water (水 shuǐ) energy of the kidneys. Then, the rest of the wood, metal and earth energy are also maximized to fulfill the coexistence and incompatibility. As a result, the change of the yin and yang can equilibrate with its polarization at maximum. Mutual changing, balancing and conflicting of yin and yang is defined as 'the ultimate extreme' (太極 tàijí).

Therefore, fire must simmer down before a practitioner reaches an auspicious (祥瑞 xiángruì) and tranquil state. A precondition of 'xin qi xia jiang' is 'quan shen fang song'. The mind can truly be quieted if the body is completely relaxed and in a deep state of rest. The reason for this is that the body and mind always interact together.

If the body is uncomfortable, then the mind is uncomfortable as well. If the mind is uncomfortable, then the body will follow suit. Just like a deep and sweet slumber can refresh the body and mind, the body will always feel more comfortable – provided the mind also gets a chance to relax in a profound manner.

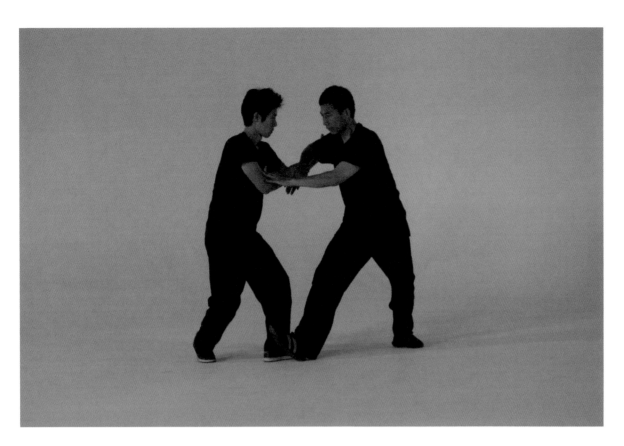

Shifu Chen Bing and I performing 'Dispersing Shadow Flower' (踩花 luàn cǎi huā) in June 2013 - Orange County, CA

12. 意守丹田 Yì Shǒu Dān Tián

Meaning

Yi: Intention **Shou:** Protect **Dan:** Red or immortal **Tian:** Field

Direct translation

Protect dantian with intention.

Practical translation

Focus on the dantian with intention and observe internally.

氣沈丹田 Qì Chén Dān Tián

Meaning

Qi: Energy **Chen:** Sink **Dan:** Red or immortal **Tian:** Field

Direct translation

Sink energy into dantian.

Practical translation

All the energy of the upper and lower body is focused and kept in the lower abdomen.

Annotation

In the direct translation, 'dan tian' is interpreted as a 'red field' because, with the exception of the heart, all of the internal organs are densely concentrated in the lower abdomen. The lower abdomen not only houses the reproductive organs, but many other organs, through which blood circulates. In ancient times, the practice of engaging the lower abdomen area was referred to as the 'medicine of the immortal' (神藥 shén yào), and the term 'elixir field' (丹田 dān tián) was later developed. If one could purify (淨化 jìng huà) the toxins of an area where a lot of blood is condensed, it would be like the immortal (神仙 shén xiān) cure. So it is referred to by that term. In traditional Chinese and Korean medicine, the dantian is also called the ocean of energy (氣海 qì hǎi). In this understanding, one could survive if one lost branches of the body such as arms and legs. However, according to traditional Chinese medicine, one could not live healthy enough without the internal organs (the five viscera and the six entrails) although advances in modern medicine have made that possible in many instances. Developing energy in the lower abdomen nourishes our vital force, providing rest to all organs and the body. Simple proof is that the elixir field is the area where our mother's womb exists and from where we are born.

'Yi shou dan tian' is simple. Breathe by directly using the navel. The navel expands with inhalation and retracts with exhalation. Thoughts sink naturally to the lower abdomen which is the 'dan tian' area. This is 'protect the elixir field by intention'. It is feasible to sense this area since the lower abdominal muscle is used directly while breathing. Novices are recommended to think that the dan tian is the entire lower abdomen in order to grasp a preliminary understanding of the concept. If 'yi shou dan tian' is accomplished, 'qi chen dan tian' should manifest naturally as the mind is followed by combining the meaning and thought once they are fulfilled. The meaning and thought is intention (意念 yì niàn) defined. Intention fluctuates always, but the mind does not.

The dan tian in Chen Family Taijiquan is not simply something to imagine or feel by the mind only. In fact it involves a very precise process that practitioners use to discover the location and physical presence of the dantian.

Within 'qi chen dan tian', there are three physical sensations to experience. They are: 'heavy' (重 zhòng), 'full' (滿 mǎn) and 'open' (開 kāi) all occurring simultaneously. If a practitioner can discover these 3 sensations, the dan tian, as required by Chen Family Taijiquan will be formed (形成 xíng chéng).

By deepening the practice, practitioners are able to discover their own experiences of dan tian clearly, and the feelings might vary. However, this sensation or experience should not fall outside of the three sensations. This is considered the correct or proper 'dan tian' according to Chen Family Taijiquan. The dan tian is located three finger joints downwards from the navel and it may vary slightly due to differing individual body types.

The Chen family created Taijiquan, and my teacher's lineage calls this 'sink down' (下沈 xià chén) - an abridged word from 'xin qi **xia** jiang' and 'qi **chen** dan tian'.

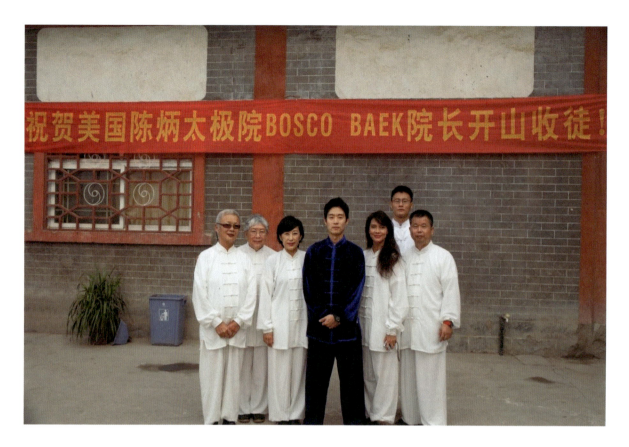

My first 6 disciples and I on October 5 2014

At Chen Bing Taiji Academy Chenjiagou Headquarters

From left, Pamela Hom, Mayanne Krech, Haeyoung Kim, me, Linda Asuma, Christopher Wang and Aaron Hong

On October 5 2014, Shifu Chen Bing and I had our disciple ceremonies in Chenjiagou. That was my teacher's grand scale disciple ceremony accepting 50 disciples and my first 6 disciples.

13. 感受呼吸 Gǎn Shòu Hū Xī

Meaning

Gan: Feel   **Shou:** Take   **Hu:** Exhale   **Xi:** Inhale

Direct translation

Feel and take exhalation and inhalation.

Practical translation

Maintain natural breathing and deeply feel as it manifests from inside.

Annotation

Try to sense the breathing when practicing Taijiquan. It should never be unnatural or laborious. It is very natural while sleeping or walking. Therefore, be aware of your breath and focus on it naturally; experience your breathing and observe it internally, as it is.

For example, most practitioners are too focused on other key disciplines while forgetting to breathe in standing post. If there is no breathing, there is no internal energy (內氣 nèi qì). When one finds and feels their breaths, concentration comes spontaneously and it is possible to achieve 'fang song'. Please keep in mind that breathing should be effortless and done around the lower abdomen area at all times.

If you observed a group of people breathing, let's say while they were lying down on a floor, you might notice that an infant or the healthier individual has deep respiration originating from the belly. Due to the lower abdominal breathing while sleeping, we refresh our energy and recover from sickness because sleeping is thought of as a characteristic of the negative which allows cultivation of energy and life force. However, nobody is conscious of breathing while fast asleep. So breathing is always natural and done from the lower abdomen all the time.

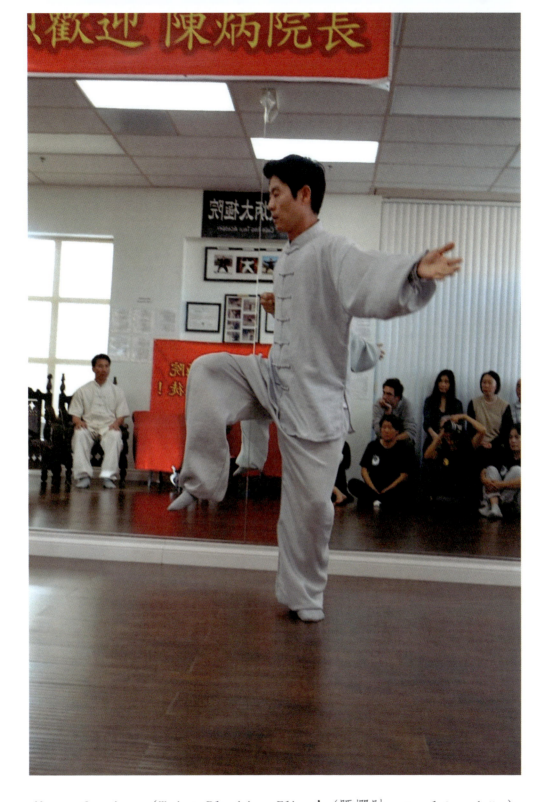

Me performing 'Waist Blocking Elbow' (腰攔肘 yāo lán zhǒu)

in Old Frame Second Road (Cannon Fist) in June 2015 - Los Angeles, CA

14. 氣貫周身 Qì Guàn Zhōu Shēn

Meaning

Qi: Energy   **Guan:** Penetrate   **Zhou:** Far and wide   **Shen:** Body

Direct translation

Penetrate energy far through the body.

Practical translation

Energy interpenetrates extensively throughout every part of the body and moves the body.

Annotation

'Qi guan zhou shen' is liberally translated as 'energy interpenetrates as one from the beginning to the end' (一氣貫通 yí qì guàn tōng) and 'the entire body is led to move by energy' (以氣運身 yǐ qì yùn shēn). There will always be three phenomenon when energy interpenetrates through the body. The first one is heat, the second is sweat, and the third is trembling (vibration). These are clear indicators that one's Taijiquan practice is progressing smoothly. If one does not experience heat or sweating, it means that there is a problem with the key disciplines in one's Taijiquan practice. The physical vibration will disappear naturally when the lower body and power (力量 lì liàng) of the body increases. The feeling can be likened to that of a worm crawling on the surface of one's skin. Swelling or numbness around the palm, accompanied by a sensation resembling the body expanding far and wide, is the sign of a revelation (發顯 fā xiǎn) of 'qi guan zhou shen'.

As it will overflow when a bowl is full of water, and a baby will walk without being taught when it is ready, energy circulation in the meridian pathways will be realized very naturally when the time is ripe. For instance, with proper training and practice the four meridians of the upper body (girdle, conception, governing and penetration-vessels) will be effortlessly full and overflow with energy; and when the four meridians of the lower body (yang-heel, yang-linking, yin-heel and yin-linking) are stimulated by 'bend the knees and relax the hips' (qu xi song kua), then the eight extraordinary channels are full of energy from practice.

It is not necessary to obstinately practice or drudgingly gain the microcosmic (小周天 xiǎo zhōu tiān) or macrocosmic orbit (大周天 dà zhōu tiān). A practitioner will self-realize such things when they are ready through in depth training.

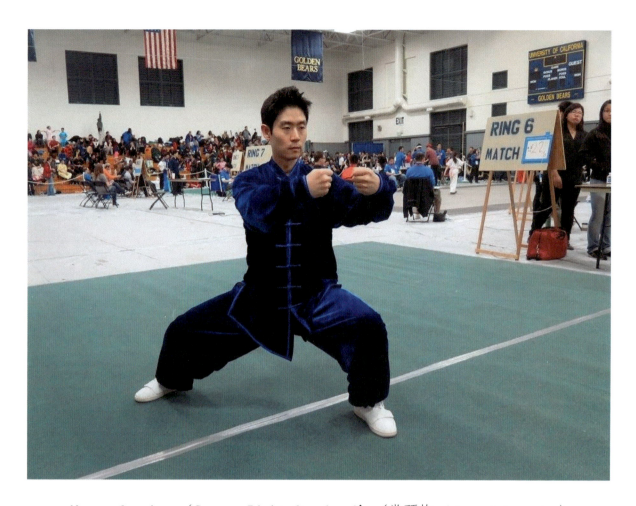

Me performing 'Cannon Right Overhead' (當頭炮 dàng tóu pào) at 24th Chinese Martial Arts Tournament (CMAT) on March 12 2016 in Berkeley, CA

15. 不丟不頂 Bù Diū Bù Dǐng

Meaning

Bu: Not   **Diu:** Lost   **Bu:** Not   **Ding:** Top or greatly

Direct translation

Not to be lost and greatly.

Practical translation

The intention and the Law of the Mind should not be overused to avoid rendering the mind too congested (停滯 ting zhì) due to too much focus on such things.

Annotation

This discipline of 'bu diu bu ding' is not only the Law of the Mind (心法 xīn fǎ), but also the Law of Intention (意念法 yì niàn fǎ). As aforementioned, the mind is the master of intention. When using intention or the Law of the Mind, it can't lose its meaning or be overly concentrated. Originally, a meaning of '頂 dǐng' was generally used as 'the crown/top of head' or 'top', but here in this sentence it is more appropriate to interpret as 'greatly'. While training the Law of

Intention and the Law of Mind, its meaning should be maintained, but not be excessive or overdone at all times. Under the right guidance from a qualified teacher, 'bu diu bu ding' will be mastered. For practice of push-hands (推手 tuī shǒu) and applications (用法 yòng fǎ), it should be applied in the same way.

When practicing the standing post, an effort is required to unearth the 9 keys of the Law of Body, and the 6 keys of the Law of Mind, which total 15 key disciplines. The standing post is like the best kind of wine (铭酒 míng jiǔ) so it becomes more mature and tasty as time goes by. As the standing post practice deepens, the reeling silk and forms will also deepen the **profound study** (功夫过硬 gōng fū guò yìng) of Taijiquan!

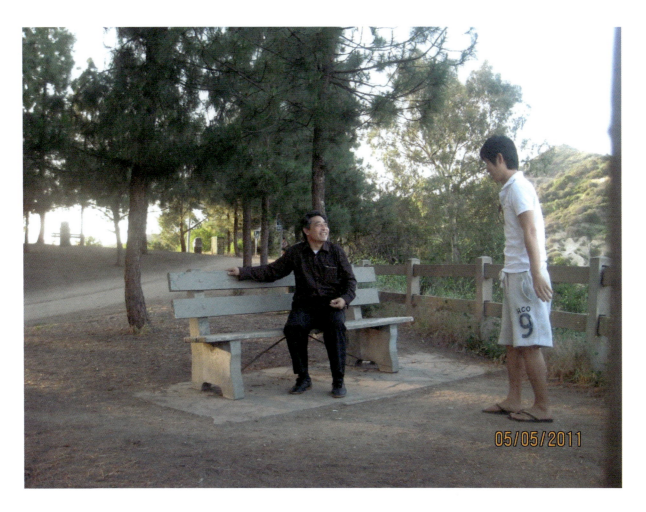

Shiye Chen Xiaoxing and I laughing in Griffith Park - Los Angeles, CA

Since 2002, I have been also studying from my teacher's second uncle Grand Master Chen Xiaoxing. His hands-on corrections helped a lot in understanding the key disciplines of Taijiquan. I call Grand Master Chen Xiaoxing and his older brother Grand Master Chen Xiaowang my 'teacher grand fathers' (師爺 shī yé) because they are my teacher's uncles as well as my teacher's teachers.

The Law of Reeling Silk (纏絲法 chán sī fǎ)

When following the Laws of Body and Mind, the upper and lower body constantly move through the elixir field (丹田 dān tián) like a coiling and spiraling thread.

This is called 'the exercise discipline of Chen Family Taijiquan' (陳氏太極拳的運動法則 chén shì tài jí quán de yùn dòng fǎ zé).

The thread (絲 sī) becomes silk (緋緞 fēi duàn).

16. 以腰爲軸 Yǐ Yāo Wéi Zhóu

Meaning

Yi: According to or by   **Yao:** Waist   **Wei:** Do, for or become   **Zhou:** Axis, axle or shaft

Direct translation

According to the waist, do as an axis.

Practical translation

All movements are initiated by the waist and body trunk becoming an axis and the hands follow the body.

Annotation

When Law of Body and Mind are maturing, eventually it is very suitable to practice the Law of Reeling Silk in Chen Family Taijiquan. The idea that the waist becomes an axis means to use the lower abdomen, the Dan Tian, as the center of movement. The lower belly and lower back becomes a spindle and the center of movement. While the front of the lower belly (elixir field: dan tian) and the lower back (life door: ming men) play a key role to move, the movement is initiated through the hip, knee and heel in the lower body – delivered through the lower back, chest, shoulder, arm and hand in the upper body, evenly and in order. This is called the Law of Reeling Silk (纏絲法 chán sī fǎ).

When becoming skillful at silk reeling, it is possible to produce the required force of Chen Family Taijiquan, which is known as the power of reeling silk (纏絲勁 chán sī jìn). It is not Chen Family Taijiquan if the Law of Reeling Silk is absent. If there is no force from reeling silk, it is not considered real power (勁 jìn) in Taijiquan.

In other words, it is not Taijiquan's hardness, softness, fastness and slowness without possessing the law and force mechanism of reeling silk. This is the major difference between Taijiquan and other practices. Without proper study of the Laws of Body and Mind, silk reeling practice might harm one's physical condition, or there will be no significant effect. The elixir field should become the center when initiating reeling silk power. This is why some Chen Family Taijiquan masters call it 'the dan tian core' (丹田核心 dān tián hé xīn).

To understand 'yi yao wei zhou' in the easiest way, grab a rope. Take the center of the rope and lift it up. The rope will wilt in half, into two parts, both dangling downwards. Slowly roll it between your thumb and fingers, to the left then to the right.

By rotating the center, the rope, in two parts, coils and spirals simultaneously. This is the easiest understanding of 'yi yao wei zhou'. Next, take the bottom and top of the rope and rotate each end in opposite directions. As it continues to rotate, the rope will become increasingly coiled and spiral into a helix. Gradually, it will thicken and densify after additional rotations. In the beginning, it starts as a supple rope, but it twists into a rigid and solid one in the end. Similarly, while the silk reeling practice opens and closes both upper and lower body continuously through 'yi yao wei zhou', the body will progressively increase in solidity and grow stronger through the force of this powerful exercise. This is the discipline detailing how the power of hardness (剛勁 gāng jìn) is produced by the power of softness (柔勁 róu jìn). At an advanced level, usually after several years when the dantian has been fully developed, it is possible to initiate the dantian from the arms, legs or in theory any part of the body. For example, the hands or legs could initiate the dantian when the inner connection of peng jin (ward-off) is being blocked by an opponent's incoming force.

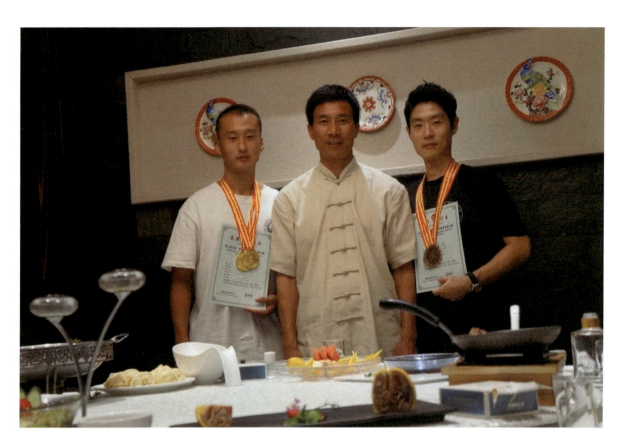

My Taiji younger brother (师弟 shī dì) Chen Chen (陈晨), Shifu Chen Bing and I in August 2015 during celebration of our medals from the 8th Jiaozuo International Taijiquan Exchange Competition

17. 胸腰折叠 Xiōng Yāo Zhé Dié

Meaning

Xiong: Chest   **Yao:** Waist   **Zhe:** Incurvate   **Die:** Fold

Direct translation

The chest and waist incurvates and folds.

Practical translation

The chest and waist folds and unfolds continuously with a connection like an ocean wave.

Annotation

'Xiong yao zhe die' is a unique Chen Family discipline that explains how the chest and waist open/close constantly while in motion and when practicing Taijiquan. The entire spine moves like an ocean wave from the neck (cervical) to the tailbone (coccyx) so that the thoracic and lumbar can repeat opening and closing via certain movements. 'Xiong yao zhe die' is feasible from the top to the bottom, from the bottom to the top, from right to left, or from left to right through physical movements and energy circulation (運身運勁 yùn shēn yùn jìn).

By deepening this principle, a motion will become smaller and more subtle. The spine will become like an elastic bamboo tree and soft as a baby's skin. In addition, a practitioner will learn how to discharge and generate power more effectively by studying this principle because it requires the whole body coordination from the movement of the spine, arms and legs all together. In Chen Family Taijiquan, the Small Frame (小架 xiǎo jià) and New Frame (新架 xīn jià) practices tend to focus on this principle.

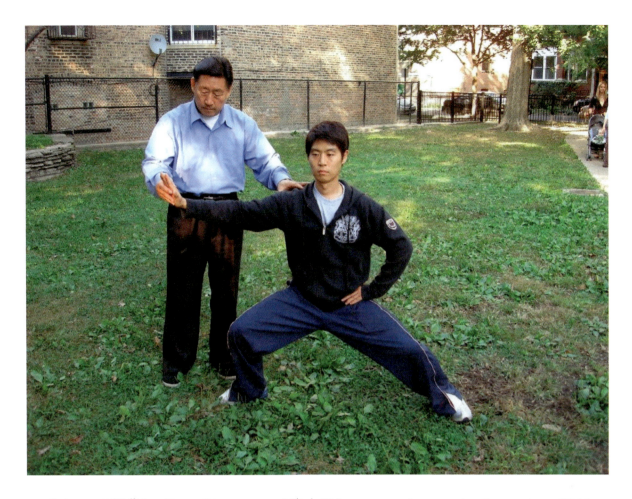

Shiye （师爷） Chen Xiaowang （陈小旺）correcting me in September 2006 - Chicago, IL

Because of my Shifu Chen Bing's arrangement, I actually had the best training seasons in my life from 2004 to 2009 while living in Chicago. It was learning from Shiye Chen Xiaoxing in March, my shifu Chen Bing in June and Shiye Chen Xiaowang in September annually in Chicago.

18. 丹田運轉 Dān Tián Yùn Zhuǎn

Meaning

Dan: Red or immortal   **Tian:** Field   **Yun:** Move   **Zhuan:** Rotate

Direct translation

Dan tian moves and rotates.

Practical translation

Dan tian moves and rotates directly internally and externally (內外 nèi wài).

Annotation

As described in 'sink energy down to elixir field' (qi chen dan tian), the dan tian in Chen Family Taijiquan is not imagined, but indeed it is actually felt. The entire lower abdomen area moves wholly with sensations of heaviness, fullness and openness within. The meridian point of the elixir field (丹田穴 dān tián xué) in the lower belly is used directly to actively move the dan tian area.

When practicing silk reeling exercise, 'dan tian yun zhuan' must always appear. The movement and rotation of the dan tian area can't be easily seen as practice deepens and skill level increases. So it is also called internal rotation of dan tian (丹田內轉 dān tián nèi zhuǎn).

Suppose there is a coin on your palm. In order to move the coin, one can do so rather naturally if the entire palm is moving. Let's say the coin represents dan tian and the palm is the lower abs, metaphorically speaking. Then, the same rule could be applied. Using only thoughts and mind is not enough to move the dan tian. We must directly initiate and physically move the entire lower abdomen while implementing the key disciplines of Taijiquan. If done correctly, the dan tian itself is moved by the entire lower abdomen.

There are three types of dan tian rotation. Dan tian moves externally and internally at the same time as the aforementioned example. The first technique is a horizontal rotation which causes dan tian to move to the left and the right. The second technique is a vertical rotation which makes the dan tian move to the front and back with an up and down method. The third technique is a combination of the horizontal and vertical dan tian rotations at once.

Everyone possesses a dan tian, but not everyone knows how to use it. The key disciplines of Chen Family Taijiquan help immensely to optimize and maximize one's dan tian. It is possible to develop your elixir field progressively by using it often.   There are no limitations for its capacity as your practice deepens.

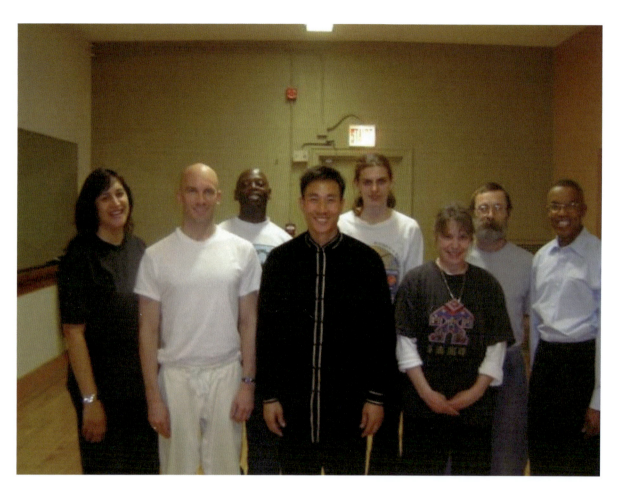

My first Chen Family Taiji group in Chicago from 2004 - 2009

19. 節節貫串 Jié Jié Guàn Chuàn

Meaning

Jie: Joint   **Jie:** Joint   **Guan:** Pass   **Chuan:** Penetrate

Direct translation

Pass and penetrate through joint by joint.

Practical translation

One by one, joint by joint, part by part and step by step, move successively and interpenetrate continuously as one.

Annotation

'Jie jie guan quan' talks about exercising the whole body in Taijiquan. Through dan tian rotation (dan tian yun zhuan), the waist moves as an axis (yi yao wei zhu) while the spine folds/unfolds (xiong yao zhe die). This occurs simultaneously, with the force mechanism of reeling silk (chan si fa) which in turn interpenetrates:

1. Heel
2. Ankle
3. Knee

4. Hip

5. Waist

6. Chest

7. Shoulder

8. Arm

9. Hand

It moves one by one, joint by joint, in order. It is better to clearly study the nine parts as shown above when practicing silk reeling and forms because that will lead to a physical understanding to help decode this principle. Theoretically speaking, the entire vertebral columns in the spine (7 cervical + 12 thoracic + 5 lumbar + 5 (fused) sacrum + 4 (fused) coccyx = 33 vertebral columns) are initiated to move gently.

More specifically, it is highly recommended to possess an awareness of three joints (parts) in the body from relaxation exercises. For instance, the arms have three joints which are the wrist, elbow and shoulder. The torso (upper body) also has three parts which are the chest, upper abdomen and lower abdomen (dan tian area) which takes control of the entire spine. The leg also has three parts which include the hip, knee and ankle to rule the entire lower body. While practicing the reeling silk exercise, commonly known as silk-reeling, although grammatically speaking, reeling silk is the proper translation from Mandarin Chinese, a practitioner should sense and feel those three parts to acquire this discipline. After cultivating sensitivity and physical feeling in each joint's motion, it is feasible to initiate every single joint and body part at once. This is the true meaning of 'jie jie guan chuan' and the core of Taijiquan exercise. Depending on a posture, it is possible to produce spiraling energy from the hand to the heel, from the heel to the crown of the head, or from the left to the right, through different forms of reeling silk in which the Law of Silk Reeling's order changes. The practitioner who truly acquires 'jie jie guan chuan' knows the essence (精髓 jīng suǐ) of Taijiquan's silk reeling core mechanism. This whole body connection and continuous movement will fiercely interpenetrate the entire body and will result in removing any blockages or foul energies.

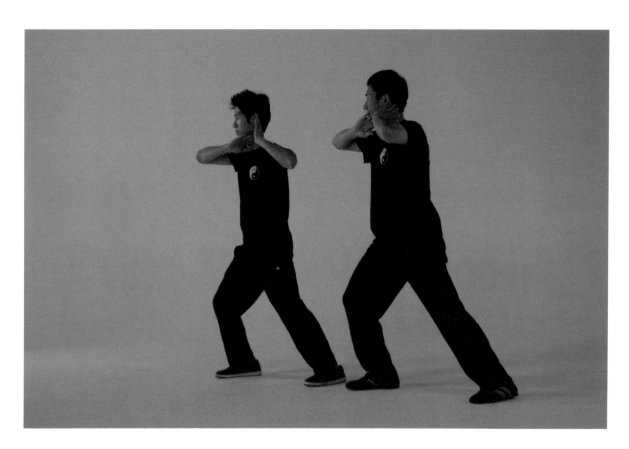

Shifu Chen Bing and I performing 'Six Sealing Four Closing' (封四閉 liù fēng sì bì) in Old Frame First Road

May 2013 - Orange County, CA

20. 意到氣到 Yì Dào Qì Dào

Meaning

Yi: Intention **Dao:** Reach **Qi:** Energy **Dao:** Reach

Direct translation

Intention reaches and then energy reaches.

Practical translation

Energy will flow where intention goes.

氣到形到 Qì Dào Xíng Dào

Meaning

Qi: Energy **Dao:** Reach **Xing:** Shape **Dao:** Reach

Direct translation

Energy reaches and then shape reaches.

Practical translation

A form is made where energy goes.

Annotation

This discipline has a lot of in depth meanings and it will be used differently given the level and quality of one's practice.

Qigong (氣功法 qì gōng fǎ), meditation (冥想 míng xiǎng), and Yoga practices share a common thread (一脈相通 yí mài xiāng tōng) between them and do not swerve off of this key principle. Intention is free and unlimited, but changes drastically. Training intention is to train mental strength (精神力 jīng shen lì). Deep concentration can render amazing effects. However there will be various drawbacks in practicing intention if there is insufficient physical preparation. Downfalls in qigong and meditation occur when intention is focused on without developing the body in a specific way first. It is because the formed 'mind' which controls intention itself is an invisible and powerful energy. Without great physical preparation of the body, the overuse of mind would be easily driven without control.

For example, let us think of an old fashioned automobile with a rusted body. How about installing an oversized and high performance engine in there? The rusted body can't handle the power (or weight) of the engine. Everyone's intention is able to develop and grow like the oversized, high performance engine. It is because there is no limitation to the use of intention and mind.

The body and frame of that car will break unless its external body force (身力 shēn lì) is already developed by specific standards to accommodate the engine. Therefore we cannot enjoy the internal mind power (心力 xīn lì) through marvelous intention due to an underdeveloped external body. This is the downfall of overdoing mental power and it will be useless (無用之物 wú yòng zhī wù) without developing the external body first. The true meaning of Taijiquan's 'balance of yin and yang' means to equally develop and harmonize the body and mind. Overtraining the body is not right and overtraining the mind is not good either. The body and mind should be practiced in a well-balanced and harmonious way. There is no point in training the Law of Mind without study or preparation of the Law of Body. This rule should be applied not only in Taijiquan, but also in Yoga, Qi Gong and other practices.

This particular discipline 'Where intention goes, then energy follows. Where energy goes, and then shape is formed.' (yi dao qi dao, qi dao xing dao)' is the discipline that combines the Law of Body and Law of Mind. If using intention correctly, energy is controllable – forms and shapes are completed. Forms of Taijiquan will change in external appearances and internal energy changes by virtue of the depth of a practitioner's study. Through the discipline of 'yi dao qi dao, qi dao xing dao', it is possible to execute energy circulation in the meridian channels (經絡運氣 jīng luò yùn qi) and to enjoy a great benefit that directly sends or stores energy where practitioners want.

For instance, it is possible to circulate energy in the meridian pathways with the key discipline of 'pass and penetrate joint by joint (jie jie guan chuan), which is:

1. Small hand pericardium(pinky finger), great foot spleen (ribs)
2. Elixir field in conception vessel (front of body)
3. Governing vessel (back of body)
4. Small intestine (back of shoulder)

when practicing silk reeling. Or, when practicing double-arm small reeling silk, it is possible to use the meridians of

1. Conception vessel to governing vessel - microcosmic orbit
2. Governing vessel to conception vessel - counter microcosmic orbit

Note: To learn more about meridian pathways, the reader should study a qualified Chinese medicine textbook.

'Yi dao qi dao, qi dao xing dao' is not just using the mind. It is to actually and very directly use the body and mind along with other key disciplines of Chen Family Taijiquan. If correctly trained in this principle, it will trigger spontaneous internal concentration and external motion which creates powerful energy circulation (運氣 yùn qi).

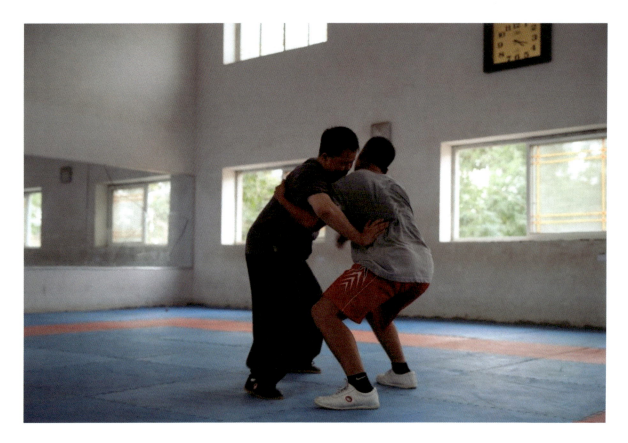

My disciple Aaron Hong and Taiji younger brother Chen Chen (陈晨 chén chén) practicing applications in free steps in October 2014 - Chenjiagou

21. 內外相合 Nèi Wài Xiāng Hé

Meaning

Nei: In   **Wai:** Out   **Xiang:** Mutual   **He:** Combine

Direct translation

Combine in and out mutually.

Practical translation

Harmonize the internal and external mutually.

周身一家 Zhōu Shēn Yì Jiā

Meaning

Zhou: Evenly, far or wide   **Shen:** Body   **Yi:** One   **Jia:** House

Direct translation

The body becomes evenly one house.

Practical translation

Move the whole body as one harmonious form.

Annotation

When practicing Chen Family Taijiquan, the mind (the internal) and the body (the external) are combined by fang song (deep and whole body relaxation). Movements of the whole body are led by the central motion of rotation of dan tian (dan tian yun zhuan). When training Taijiquan, the body and mind (心身 xīn shēn) should be harmonized while the arms and legs should be led as one by the center of dan tian rotation. This discipline requires all of the previous ones; Law of Body, Law of Mind and the Law of Reeling Silk. It requires constant work and practice.

When moving the body, the mind moves with it. All ceases when stopped and stationary. All arises when starting and moving. When one part moves, all parts move. When one part stops, all parts stop. One's Taijiquan form becomes graceful, beautiful, elegant, harmonized and powerful. Only a practitioner who has reached an advanced level of study knows the secret (奧義 ào yì) of this discipline.

The Four Major Characteristics
(四大特點 sì dà tè diǎn)

The 4 significant features (特徵 tè zhēng) of Chen Family Taijiquan always appear when the Laws of Body, Mind and Reeling Silk are harmonized.

They are very important guidelines (指針 zhǐ zhēn) of Taijiquan practice.

22. 剛柔并(相)濟 Gāng Róu Bīng(Xiàng) Jǐ

Meaning

Gang: Hard   **Rou:** Soft   **Bing (Xiang):** Mutual   **Ji:** help, cross or beneficial

Direct translation

Help the hard and soft mutually.

Practical translation

Harmonize the hardness and softness (to be beneficial to each other).

快慢相間 Kuài Màn Xiàng Jiàn

Meaning

Kuai: Fast   **Man:** Slow   **Xiang:** Mutual   **Jian:** Mix, ~ between, or trap

Direct translation

Mix the fast and the slow mutually.

Practical translation

Change/Mix the fastness and slowness.

Annotation

The original Chen Family Taijiquan requires hardness, softness, fastness and slowness to mutually cross and blend together. The slowness and softness are the negative '陰 yīn' and the fastness and hardness are the positive '陽 yáng'. This discipline implies the balance and change of Ying and Yang in Chen Family Taijiquan. As aforementioned, the meaning of the ultimate extreme (太极 tài jí) is the harmony (造化 zào huà), change (變化 biàn huà) and balance (平衡 píng héng) of the negative (yin) and the positive (yang). If these are not maintained, it violates the rule of Taijiquan. This key 'the fastness and slowness mutually mix and exist (gang rou bing (xiang) ji, kuai man xiang jian)' must appear when training Chen Family Taijiquan forms. Just practicing slowly or softly is only half of Taijiquan and will not seize (掌握 zhǎng wò) the balance of ying and yang (陰陽變化 yīn yáng biàn huà) which Taijiquan strives towards.

As there are inconsistencies in human emotion, energy shares the same characteristics. While implementing the key disciplines of Taijiquan, the internal energy circulation can adapt against the external force.

For instance, the elixir field can internally circulate its energy slowly although an external form discharges power in fast and hard motions. In other words, in possessing the key principles, the external power will also be dexterously adaptable depending on one's energy capacity and application.

Let us contemplate how Yang Lu Chan, the founder of Yang Family Taijiquan earned the title of 'Yang the Invincible' (楊無敵 yáng wú dí). How could he defeat many different styles of martial artists by just utilizing the slow motions for self defense? Before becoming the founder of Yang Family Taiijquan, Yang himself was a master of Chen Family Taijiquan in the eldest (嫡統 dí tǒng) and direct descendant lineage in the Chen family. In other words, he achieved a superhuman level of exquisite art (入神 rù shén) of Taijiquan and realized the discipline of 'harmonize and cross the hardness and softness mutually' (gang rou bing (xiang) ji), and 'mix and trap a change between the fastness and slowness' (kuai man xiang jian). Through the key principles of Taijiquan, Yang was able to change fluidly and fight freely by using his reaction and energy against his opponent's motion/speed.

Taijiquan is not always slow. If an opponent is fast or slow, then one should move accordingly depending on a situation by using reeling silk force. In the concept of Taijiquan's combat, the hardness, softness, fastness and slowness change quickly and deftly and are applied freely against force and applications along with good timing and speed.

In general, Taijiquan's most famous practical methods are slowness and softness (慢柔 màn róu). They are just the tools to maximize and increase one's sensitivity (感覺 gǎn jué) so that one can take control of their body and realize energy circulation. Having slowness and softness are truly beneficial to build up a healthy body for well-being (健身 jiàn shēn) and a great Taiji body structure. Therefore, Taijiquan has the nick name (別稱 bié chēng) "fist of the sensitivity fist" (感覺拳 gǎn jué quán).

After mastering 'slowness and softness', one must enter through the door to fastness and hardness (剛快 gāng kuài). The practice of 'fastness and hardness' should retain the key points that render the same energy flow and body control from mastering the sensations in 'slowness and softness'. In fact, it is possible to maintain the same conditions in reeling silk force through fast and hard motions only if a great foundation from slowness and softness has been achieved. Later, there is no boundary between the hardness and softness or fastness and slowness in applications. Please refine meticulously the fundamentals and weak parts of your forms because perfecting basics is the best way to enlighten Taiji's practical methods. You will become the divine skill as much as you deepen the basics.

The ultimate goal of Taijiquan practice is to combine and unite the negative (yin) and the positive (yang). This implies endless change in the yin and yang whenever a practitioner wants to change.

Please just keep in mind that hardness, softness, fastness and slowness (剛柔快慢 gāng róu kuài màn), without the force and Law of Reeling Silk is not Taijiquan. Without deepening the key disciplines of Chen Family Taijiquan, it will just be another empty practice. The existence of these key disciplines makes a clear distinction between Taijiquan and other practices.

Taijiquan is a delicate and systematic practice for well-being and self defense. However, that does not mean it is to be strictly in slow motion. Because there are very few successors (傳人 chuan rén) who learned from the birth place of Taijiquan, it is common to see the simplified and modern styles of Taijiquan, which are not authentic.

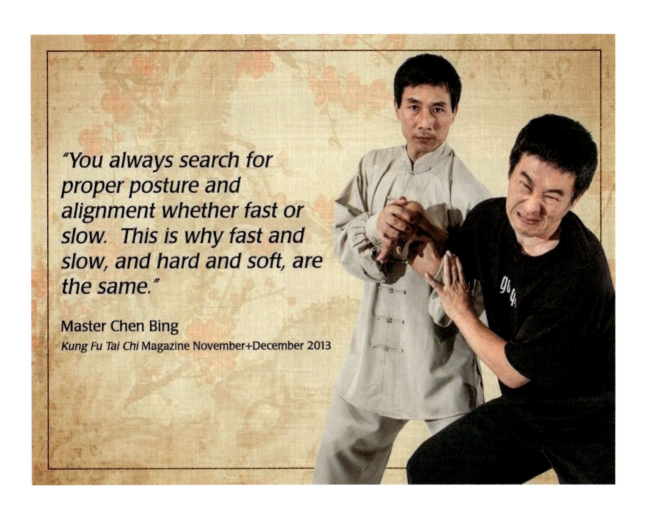

"You always search for proper posture and alignment whether fast or slow. This is why fast and slow, and hard and soft, are the same."

Master Chen Bing
Kung Fu Tai Chi Magazine November+December 2013

23. 蓄發相變 Xù Fā Xiāng Biàn

Meaning

Xu: Cultivate   **Fa:** Discharge   **Xiang:** Mutual   **Bian:** Change

Direct translation

Cultivating and discharging mutually change.

Practical translation

Saving energy on the inside and discharging energy to the outside change mutually (in motion).

Annotation

Saving energy is called 'xu qi (蓄氣 xù qì)' and discharging energy is called 'fa qi (發氣 fā qì)'. Saving force is called 'xu jin (蓄勁 xù jìn)' and discharging force is called 'fa jin (發勁 fā jìn)'. Energy (qi) itself is very weak and can be easily altered by internal change and stimulation. For instance, energy will be active if the body and mind are comfortable or when one is experiencing happiness. However, energy will be inactive if the body and mind are uncomfortable or when one is feeling melancholy.

If the focus of the Law of Mind (調心 tiáo xīn – 神 shén, spirit), energy of the breathing (調息 tiáo xī – 氣 qì, energy) from dan tian, posture of the Law of Body (調身 tiáo shēn – 精 jīng, essence) are united, energy (氣 qì) can be developed and refined into force (勁 jìn).

'Jin' is the condensed and concentrated energy (qi) which is not easily shattered.

By the theory of yin and yang, saving energy is 'yin' and shooting energy is 'yang'. While practicing Taijiquan, this 'xu fa xiang bian' always changes and complements (補完 bǔ wán) each other.

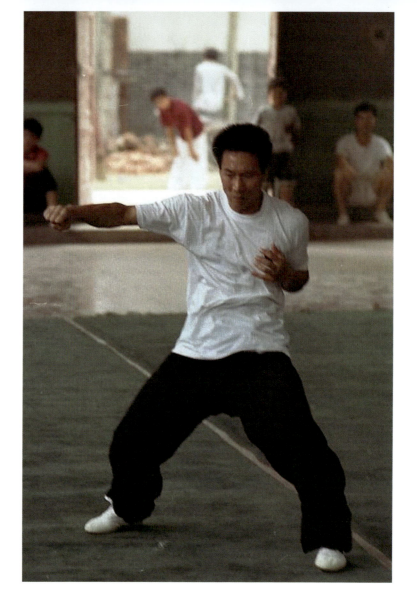

Shifu Chen Bing's 'Hide Hand Forearm Fist'

(掩手肱拳 yǎn shǒu gōng quán) – August 2002 in Chenjiagou

My teacher's explosive power is really fierce not only in demonstration but also in application. When I asked him about the secret of powerful explosion, he happily smiled and answered 'it is fang song!'

24. 鬆活彈抖 Sōng Huó Tán Dǒu

Meaning

Song: Relax **Huo:** Alive **Tan:** Elasticity **Dou:** Vibrate

Direct translation

Be relaxed, alive, elastic and vibrating.

Practical translation

It requires reaching a state of relaxation, being alive, having elasticity and vibrating when practicing.

Annotation

This key discipline indicates all requirements of Taijiquan practice. 'Relaxing and alive' (song huo) originates from the condition of deep relaxation (fang song) of the body and mind (心身 xīn shēn), which already is full of vital energy (活氣 huó qì). 'Tan' means elasticity of the body and it has a rubber like characteristic during the moment of discharging force. 'Dou' means the natural vibration of the body after discharging force (發勁 fā jìn).

'Song huo tan dou' draws a distinction between Chen Family Taijiquan and other styles of Taijiquan. It is not hard to achieve 'relaxing' (song), but 'being alive, elastic and vibrating' (huo, tan, dou) requires a lot of practice. More specifically, elasticity and natural vibration (tan dou) are a very unique and pure mark (純粹 chún cuì) of excellence (精華 jīng huá) in Chen Family Taijiquan when compared to other Taiji styles.

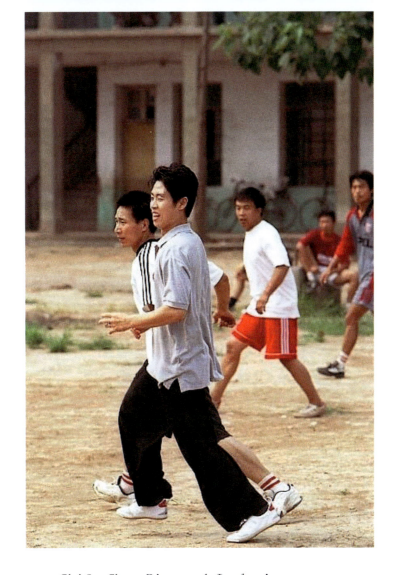

Shifu Chen Bing and I playing soccer

photo taken in August 2002 in Chenjiagou

25. 外形走弧線 Wài Xíng Zǒu Hú Xiàn

Meaning

Wai: External **Xing:** Form **Zhou:** Go **Hu:** Circle **Xian:** Line

Direct translation

It goes in a circular line in an external form.

Practical translation

The external form of the body always draws a circular line and circular movements (圓運動 yuán yùn dòng).

內勁走旋 Nèi Jìn Zǒu Luó Xuán

Meaning

Nei: Internal **Jin:** Force **Zhou:** Go **Luo:** Spiral **Xuan:** Rotate

Direct translation

The internal force rotates in a spiral line.

Practical translation

The internal force of reeling silk movement is a route that always runs a helix shape and rotates in a circle.

Annotation

During practice of Taijiquan, the external body's appearance should have a round look about it (or sometimes an ellipse) and circular motion in exercise. The internal pathway of reeling silk is a spiral and coiling shape which is a helix and can make infinite orbits of movement. The power and principles of circular motion is found in life. It is found in a tornado (颱風 tái fēng) and the wheels of cars. The tornado powerfully rotates and swirls. Its vortex rampages and passes through everything. Car wheels are round. The rotation of a wheel absorbs the power of the engine and delivers motion to the car's body. All of these come from principles of circular motion. The principles of spiral and coiling are also interesting. The DNA's structure in the human body is a double-helix (二重螺線 èr chóng luó xiàn) which stabilizes the balances of the body. So, the helix is the order of nature.

There will never be straight motions (直線 zhí xiàn), only circular movements. The reeling of silk has no certain angle to abstrusely (奧妙 ào miào) make spiral and coiling movements which constantly rotate and move inside the body. The reeling silk practice of a novice is insignificant, but later it will appear like the power of a tornado that swirls and sweeps through the entire body.

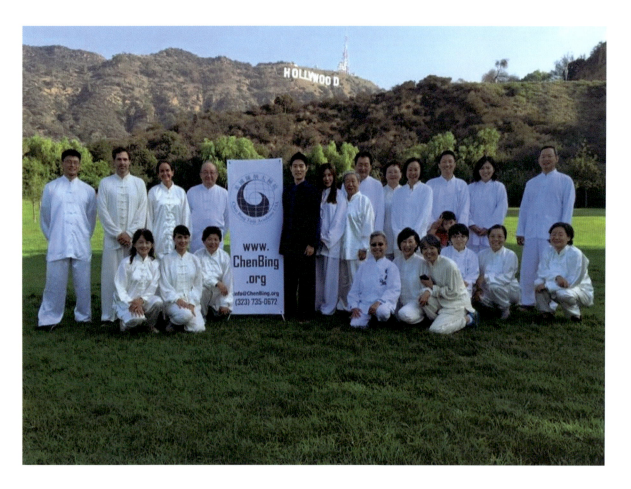

Chen Bing Taiij Academy USA in Los Angeles, CA

Photo taken in October 2015 for the Guinness Book of World Records

for the largest martial arts display (multiple venues)

General Terms in Chinese Culture

老师 lǎo shī

This means 'old teacher'. The default title is to address a teacher of any kind. It can be a teacher in an academic school, fine arts or any sport. It can be broadened in use to address an expert in any field. In fact, the word 'lao' means basically 'old', but its actual meaning is to express 'experienced and skillful' as well in phrases and sentences. Therefore, a proper understanding of 'lao shi' is an experienced teacher.

师父 shī fu

This means 'teacher father'. This is typically used in martial arts, craft or artisan apprenticeship. It denotes close family by blood or surrogate relationship. It is often misused outside Asia as Master.

师傅 shī fu

This vocabulary is the most confusing one to foreigners because it is exactly the same pronunciation as the aforementioned '师父 shī fu'. Yet, a word 'fu' is different. It indicates 'teacher craftsman' which is usually associated with professionals. It can be used to address any professional such as chef, professor, taxi driver, engineer, musician, master mechanic or master craftsman. In broad usage, 'laoshi' is only for those who are recognized as a great professional.

学生 xué sheng

This means 'study student'. It is usually associated with the typical normal student. They are free to leave and not restricted to learn any studies or practices.

徒弟 tú dì

This means 'group (same kind) brother'. It is only used for those who have a master teacher for life and have had a disciple ceremony to be recognized as a successor from a certain lineage holder in traditional practices. They are very restricted to learn any practices other than their arts. This term is broadly used for Chinese martial arts, music and craftsmanship.

弟子 dì zǐ

This means 'brother son'. It is usually used for a sincere student in any field. It is also a synonym of disciple.

师兄 shī xiōng

This means 'teacher older brother'. It is used for older or earlier accepted male disciples. For disciples in the same year who are accepted, it goes by age. But it will follow this rule by an acceptance year. For example, a person who became a disciple in 2008 and is 40 years old must call 'older brother' for the person who became a disciple in 2007 and is now 29 year old. This is classical Chinese culture.

师姐 shī jiě

This means 'teacher older sister'. It is used for older or earlier accepted female disciples.

师弟 shī dì

This means 'teacher younger brother'. It is used for younger or later accepted male disciples.

师妹 shī mèi

This means 'teacher younger sister'. It is used for younger or later accepted female disciples.

师母 shī mǔ

This means 'teacher mother' which indicates a master teacher's wife. In Chinese tradition, disciples should respect shifu's wife as equal to shifu.

师祖 shī zǔ

This means 'teacher ancestor'. It is normally used for a level of great grand father in a lineage.

师爷 shī yé

This means 'teacher grand father'. It is typically used for a teacher's male teacher such as uncle.

师奶 shī nǎi

This means 'teacher grand mother' which is typically used for a teacher's female relative such as an aunt.

师叔 shī shū

This means 'teacher uncle' which is typically used for a teacher's male cousin.

师姑 shī gū

This means 'teacher aunt' which is typically used for a teacher's female cousin or family member.

大師 dà shī

This means 'big (great) teacher' which is typically used for an internationally well-known teacher in any field.

高手 gāo shǒu

This means 'high hand' which is typically used for an expert, a master craftsman or an artisan in any field.

掌门人 zhǎng mén rén

This means 'palm gate person' which is typically used for a person who represents or is in charge of a school of martial arts, or a leader of a religious practice or academic field.

拜师式 bài shī shì

This means 'bow teacher ceremony'. It is a word for the discipleship ceremony. This is the ceremony where disciples take an oath to make a lifetime commitment to their art.

General Terms in Western Terms

Student

It is pretty much as same as Chinese culture. It is broadly used for those who learn anything.

Disciple

It is a more rarely used word for a student. Christianity recalls the 12 disciples.

Instructor

This refers to someone who teaches a specific skill. Sometimes it is used for school teacher or university professor.

Teacher

It is a person who teaches at a school, academy or similar institution as a job.

Master

This is a title created by Westerners in order to replace a word of '高手 gāoshǒu' which means 'high hand' or '师傅 shīfu' which means 'teacher artisan'. In Western countries, it is a substitute and is intended to express a master craftsman, artisan and Master in a specific field.

Grand Master

It is another Western term to replace the title of 'big (great) teacher' (大師 dà shī) and 'palm gate person' (掌门人 zhǎng mén rén) who can represent or be in charge of a school of martial arts, or a leader of a religious or academic field.

Chen Family Taijiquan Tree of Bosco Baek in USA

Chen Bu (1st generation of the Chen family)
⇩
Chen Wangting (9th generation of the Chen family, the Taijquan creator)
⇩
Chen Changxing (14th generation of the Chen family)
⇩
Chen Fake (17th generation of the Chen family)
⇩
Chen Xiaowang and Chen Xiaoxing (19th generation of the Chen family)
⇩
Chen Bing (20th generation of the Chen family)
⇩
Bosco Baek (21st generation of the Chen family)
⇩

First 6 Disciples (2014): Pam Hom, Mayanne Krech, Haeyoung Kim, Aaron Hong, Linda Asuma, Christopher Wang

Second 4 Disciple (2015): Austin Kim, Christopher Soule, Michael Manfredo, Lauren Chee

Third 10 Disciples (2017): Mija Park, Randall Krause, Midori Simovich, Atsuko Zama, Gin Kim, Sasan Jahan-Parwar, Stefanos Kafatos, Kiho Hong, Hyunmi Ahn, Seungjae Lee

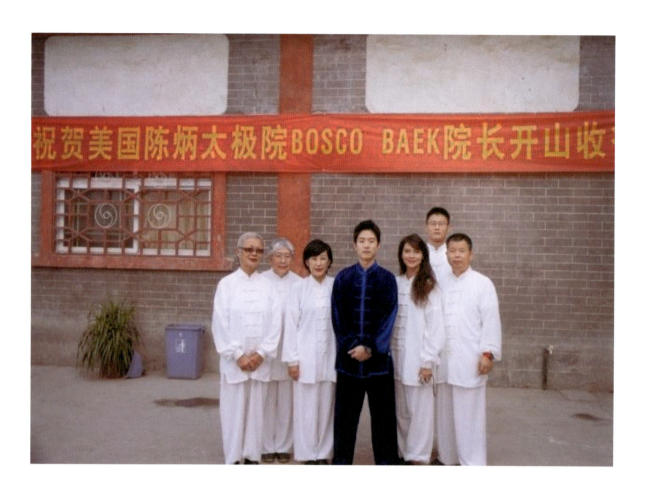

October 5, 2014 First Disciples of Master Bosco Baek in Chenjiagou

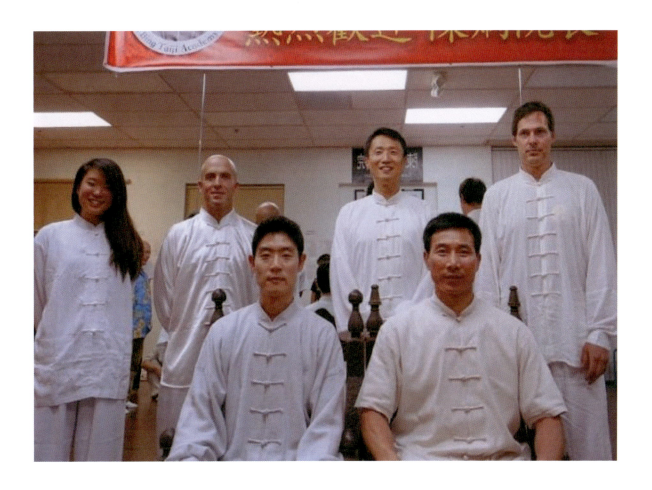

June 18, 2015 Second Disciples of Master Bosco Baek in Los Angeles

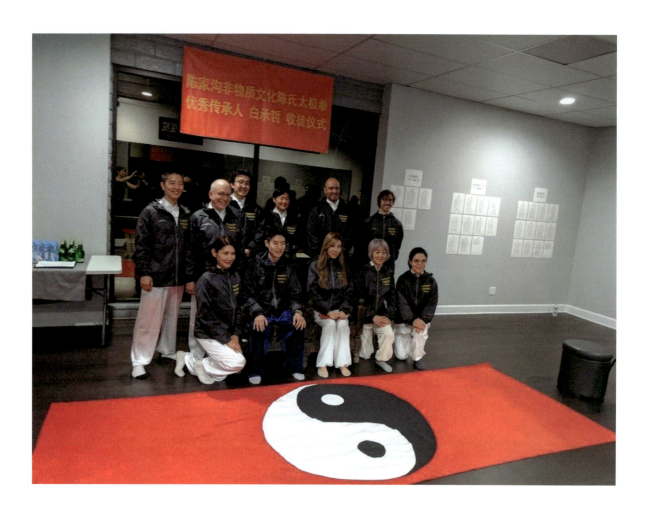

May 12, 2017 Third Disciples of Master Bosco Baek in Los Angeles

Additional Writing by Bosco Baek

Baek, Bosco. (2009). Finding Fang Song. *Inside Kung-Fu*. Vol. 37, No. 2. 70-73.

Baek, Bosco. (2009). Chen Family 5 Kinds of Push-Hands. *Inside Kung-Fu*. Vol. 37, No. 8. 52-55.

Baek, Bosco. (2010). Refreshing the Spine. *Kung Fu Tai Chi*. March/April. 10-13.

Baek, Bosco. (2011). Three Dantian Rotation Techniques in Chen Taiji. *The Journal of Asian Martial Arts*. Volume 20 Number 3. 62-85.

All copyrights (著作權 zhù zuò quán) belong to Bosco Baek of Chen Bing Taiji Academy USA.

Any reproduction, use, distribution without the explicit consent of the author will be punishable by law.

www.ChenBing.org

Printed in Great Britain
by Amazon